T0093431

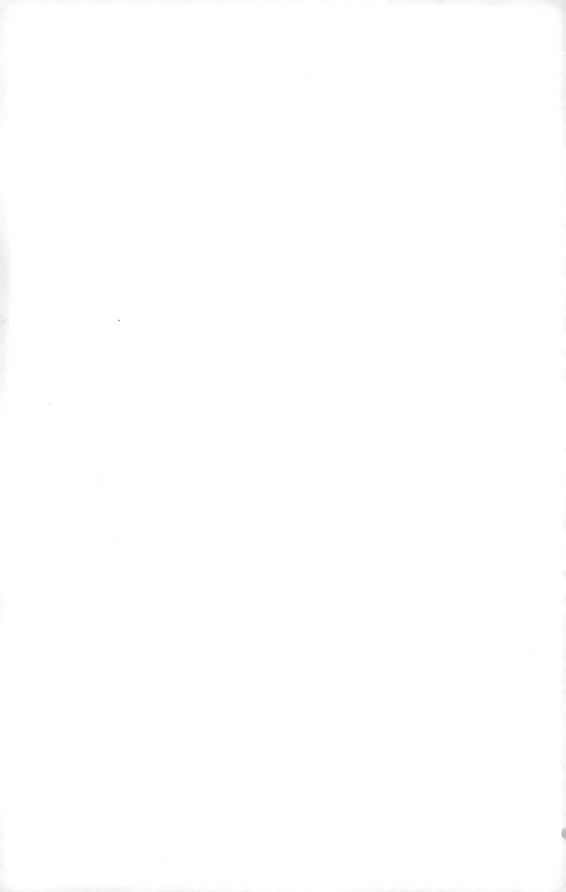

Basic Surgical Skills

An easy-to-follow, step-by-step guide to the most useful surgical skills from knot tying to simple procedures. Illustrated with colour photographs and video clips to demonstrate techniques, this book makes these practical skills as clear and easy to follow as possible.

Including coverage of surgical instruments, wound management and suturing, and minor surgical procedures, it also explains how to use these essential surgical skills to make the most of a surgical placement. Healthcare students or junior professionals undertaking a placement in surgery or emergency medicine will feel confident and capable and able to take an active role in surgical placements. Learning basic surgical skills is important for such placements, as well as for undertaking exams such as the Membership of the Royal College of Surgeons (MRCS).

Expert videos, guided by the author, are included with the book and can be accessed through www.routledge.com/9781032423265.

Basic Surgical Skills

An Illustrated Guide

Graeme M Downes

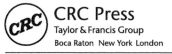

CRC Press
Taylor & Francis Group
Boca Raton New York London

CRC Press is an imprint of the
Taylor & Francis Group, an **informa** business

First edition published 2023
by CRC Press
6000 Broken Sound Parkway NW, Suite 300, Boca Raton, FL 33487-2742

and by CRC Press
4 Park Square, Milton Park, Abingdon, Oxon, OX14 4RN

CRC Press is an imprint of Taylor & Francis Group, LLC

© 2023 Taylor & Francis Group, LLC

ISBN: 978-1-032-42329-6 (hbk)
ISBN: 978-1-032-42326-5 (pbk)
ISBN: 978-1-003-36228-9 (ebk)

DOI: 10.1201/b23298

Typeset in Minion
by SPi Technologies India Pvt Ltd (Straive)

Access the Support Material: www.routledge.com/9781032423265

For my fiancée, Serena, whose support and encouragement made this book possible.
For Colette Davey, who fought to get me into surgical training.
For all those who have taken the time to offer training and advice during my career.

Contents

List of videos

Acknowledgements

Howard Chu, for the chapter on Surgical Placement.

Rituja Kamble, for the chapters on Local Anaesthesia, Wound Debridement and Cyst Excision.

Author bio

Graeme M Downes completed a medical degree at Imperial College London, having been awarded a scholarship. Following his foundation training in Plymouth, UK, he completed three years as a General Duties Medical Officer with the British Army, deploying in the UK and overseas. After coming second in national selection, he is now completing Core Surgical Training with the intention of applying for Plastic Surgery training.

He maintains a focus on education, running national training courses and tutoring for an MRCS revision company.

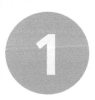

1 Introduction

Graeme M Downes

In this book we will be covering the most useful basic surgical skills, from knot tying to simple procedures. By understanding these techniques students and junior healthcare professionals will be able to take a more active and involved role in their placements and rotations. This will be covered in more detail in the final chapter, but a good grasp of these skills will enable you to demonstrate them during placements and will put you in a better position to learn more advanced techniques from your supervisors.

For those who are planning to pursue a surgical career, these basic skills will be essential throughout your training and beyond. Passing the MRCS exam is a confirmation of the skills you have developed in your early training and the basic practical knowledge you have gained. By understanding the techniques and practising them on placements you will be well placed to tackle the surgical skill station.

The skills we will be covering in this text are broadly applicable to other specialties outside surgery. Suturing and wound management skills are crucial in specialties such as emergency medicine, anaesthetics and primary care as well as for anyone wanting to undertake remote, expedition or pre-hospital work.

Throughout this book we will be making use of colour photographs utilising porcine tissue for maximum fidelity, to make these practical skills as clear and easy to follow as possible. There is no substitute for getting hands-on experience, but this guide will equip you with a sound understanding to enable you to have confidence to practise these skills.

DOI: 10.1201/b23298-1

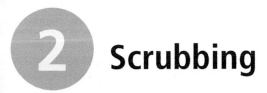

2 Scrubbing

Graeme M Downes

Ignaz Semmelweis (1818–1865) was one of the earliest proponents of effective hand hygiene. Working in obstetrics in Vienna, he made the case for hand washing which led to a reduction in perinatal infections. Semmelweis' observations could not be explained by the scientific theory of the time, and it was not until the acceptance of the germ theory of Louis Pasteur (1822–1895) that there was an explanation. These ideas were expanded by Joseph Lister (1827–1912) and the practice of antiseptic surgery was described in his 1867 *Antiseptic Principle in the Practice of Surgery*. It was because of these early proponents of asepsis that we now practise rigorous surgical hand washing and the donning of personal protective equipment.

Before starting to scrub, ensure that you have selected an appropriately sized gown pack and gloves and that these are open and ready to be donned. A mask and head covering should be worn. Depending on the operation, it may be that you choose to put on eye protection.

The first stage in preparing for surgery is to clean your hands. The first scrub of the day should be a 'social wash' where the hands are washed and a scrub brush and finger pick used to remove gross contamination.

The surgical scrub is then started: this is a seven-step process that is intended to ensure that all areas of the hands and wrists are cleaned. This is carried out with a surgical hand wash such as chlorhexidine or an iodine containing wash. It is important to ensure that the hands are held above the levels of the elbows throughout these steps.

You should first open your gown pack without touching the inner surfaces before opening a correctly sized pack of gloves using a non-touch method.

Your first hand scrub of the day should utilise a scrub brush before starting the steps detailed below.

DOI: 10.1201/b23298-2

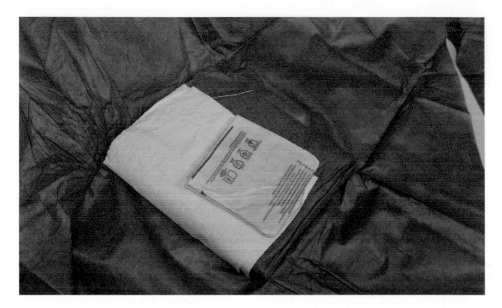

Figure 2.1 Prepare your gown and gloves before starting to scrub.

The seven-step World Health Organization technique

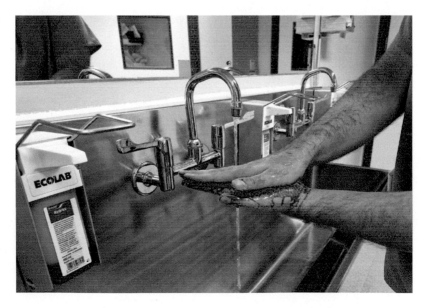

Figure 2.2 Rub your hands palm to palm.

Start by turning the tap to a suitable temperature and wetting your hands and forearms. Apply surgical scrub to your hands and rub palm to palm.

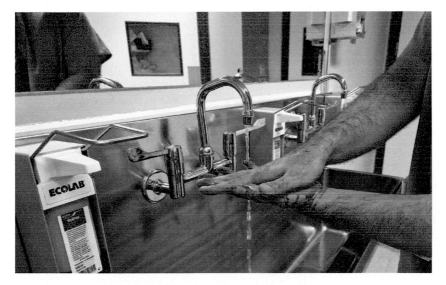

Figure 2.3 Rub your hands palm to palm with fingers interlaced.

Now rub your palms together with interlaced fingers, ensuring good coverage of the surgical scrub.

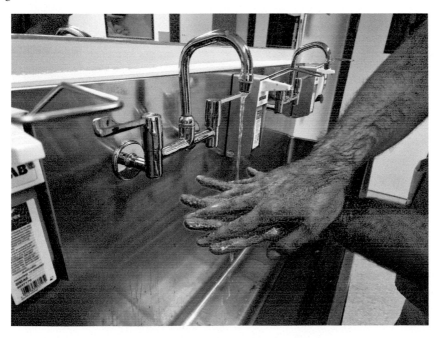

Figure 2.4 Rub your hands palm to dorsum with fingers interlaced.

Rub your right palm over the dorsum of your left hand interlacing your fingers, then swap hands.

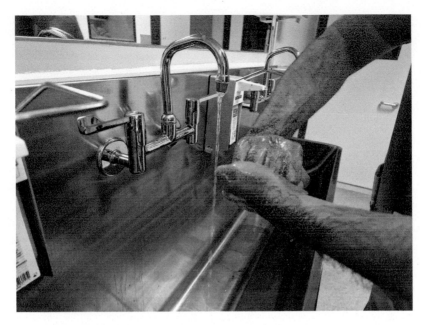

Figure 2.5 Rub your hooked fingers together.

Hook your fingers together and rub the dorsum of the fingers against the palms.

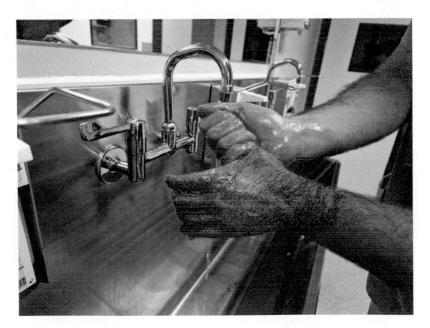

Figure 2.6 Wash your thumbs.

Grasp your left thumb in your right hand and scrub in a rotational manner, then swap hands.

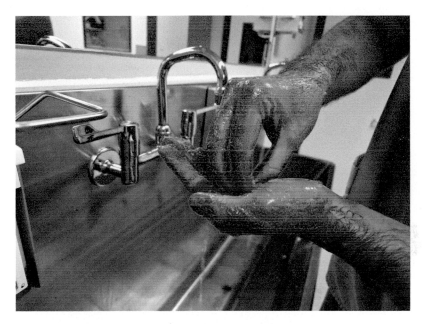

Figure 2.7 Rub your fingertips in your palm.

Dispense more soap into your left palm and rub your right fingers in it, then swap hands.

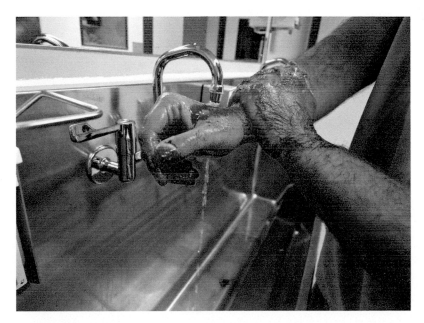

Figure 2.8 Wash your forearms.

Now use your left palm to scrub your right wrist to mid forearm, then swap hands.

Repeat the above steps but only scrub to the wrist, then turn off the tap with the elbow levers and dry your hands with sterile towels from the gown pack. You should follow your local policy on the duration of hand washing, but it should be an absolute minimum of two minutes.

The next step is for you to pick up the sterile gown and put your arms inside, ensuring that your hands do not come out of the ends of the sleeve.

At this stage you will need someone to assist you with securing the gown at the neck and waist.

Then put the gloves on, again ensuring your clean hands do not become exposed to the environment.

Once this is done, hand the tag at the front of the gown to a member of the theatre team and turn in place to wrap the waist tie in a sterile fashion before tying it yourself.

You are now fully protected to be involved in surgery!

3 Basic surgical instruments

Graeme M Downes

A knowledge of surgical instruments, including their names and uses, is crucial for efficient surgical care. Being able to select the most appropriate instrument enables you to use the most effective tool for the desired therapeutic outcome. The ability to request the correct instrument will also enable any operative case to run more efficiently and reduce the task load on you as an operator.

I am grateful for the assistance of Bailey Instruments Ltd for providing images for this chapter.

The scalpel

When choosing the right scalpel to make your incision, the first consideration is the type of handle to mount your blade on. The two most common handles are explored here.

The first is the flat handle. There are variations on this type that are numbered, like the number 4 handle pictured below. This handle is stable when making linear excisions and prevents any rolling during use. This is particularly useful when there is a preference for straight incisions and reduces the chance of slipping when the handle is wet.

The other commonly used handle is the rounded or hexagonal handle, such as the Barron handle. This is named after John N Barron, founding member of the British Association of Plastic Surgeons and later president of the subsequent organisation, the British Association of Plastic Reconstructive and Aesthetic Surgeons. As expected from the name, this handle is commonly used for incisions of the skin. The shape of the handle allows the blade to be angled and moved more easily, allowing for complex, non-linear incisions.

DOI: 10.1201/b23298-3

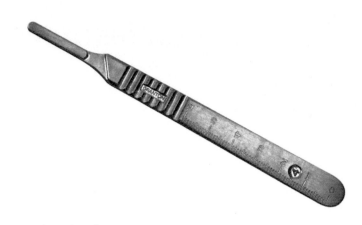

Figure 3.1 A number 4 handle.

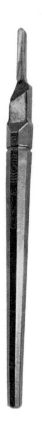

Figure 3.2 Barron handle.

Blades

Each blade is designed for a specific application and so selecting the correct one is important. The most commonly used blades for basic surgical skills are Numbers 10, 20, 12 and 15.

The 10 blade is a good general-purpose blade that has a broad cutting curve and is used for making linear incisions; the 20 is very similar in shape but larger and so is better for large linear incisions. These blades are commonly used for incisions over a subcutaneous lesion that is being excised or for gaining access to a body cavity.

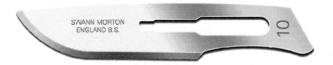

Figure 3.3 Number 10 blade.

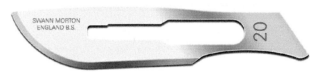

Figure 3.4 Number 20 blade.

The 12 blade is an exaggeratedly curved blade with the cutting surface on the inside of the curve. It is used for cutting stiches or drain ties.

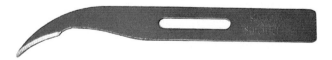

Figure 3.5 Number 12 blade.

The number 15 blade has a small, angled blade and is ideal for making precise and non-linear incisions. It is commonly used for excisions of cutaneous lesions.

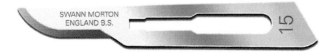

Figure 3.6 Number 15 blade.

Forceps

Forceps are instruments used to grasp tissues. There are two broad groups – toothed and non-toothed – and there are variations of each type.

Toothed forceps have a point on the tip in order to grasp tissue: this is used for grasping skin where any crushing would be inappropriate.

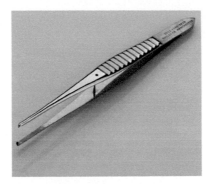

Figure 3.7 Gillies forceps – a type of toothed forceps.

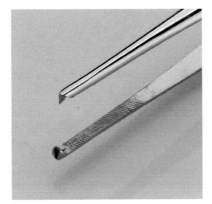

Figure 3.8 The toothed end of the forceps.

Non-toothed forceps have flat ends that are used to grasp tissues without the risk of puncturing, particularly delicate visceral tissues such as vascular structures or bowel.

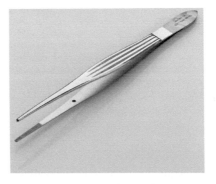

Figure 3.9 McIndoe forceps – a type of non-toothed forceps.

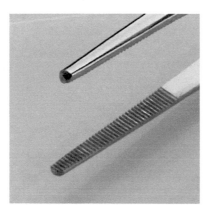

Figure 3.10 The flat end of the forceps.

Forceps, such as those above, should be held in a similar way to a pen, as demonstrated below.

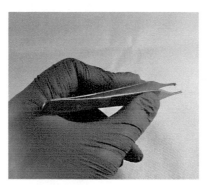

Figure 3.11 How to correctly hold forceps.

There are various clips used to hold tissues or equipment that are also termed forceps, such as artery forceps or bone forceps.

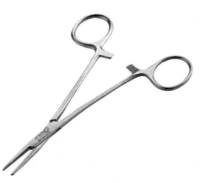

Figure 3.12 Halstead artery forceps.

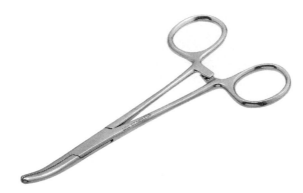

Figure 3.13 Spencer Wells forceps.

Instruments with finger spaces, such as artery forceps and scissors, should be held with half the distal phalanx of the thumb and the distal phalanx of the ring finger, leaving your index and middle fingers free to stabilise the instrument. The correct handling will be seen in later chapters where we will be looking at them in use. Knowing how the instruments are meant to be handled will make you look more professional and skilled on your placements.

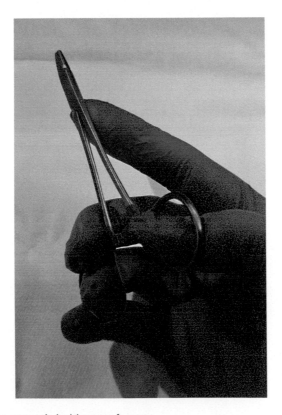

Figure 3.14 How to correctly hold artery forceps.

Needle holders

Needle holders are similar to artery forceps but are specifically designed for holding and manipulating needles during suturing. They can be distinguished by the cross-hatched pattern on the blades.

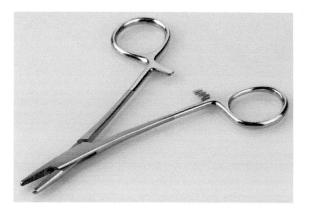

Figure 3.15 Mayo needle holders.

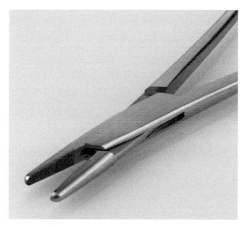

Figure 3.16 Close up of Mayo needle holders – take note of the cross-hatched pattern.

Scissors

There are different types of straight and curved scissors of various sizes. Heavier scissors are useful for cutting dressings, for example, whereas smaller scissors are used for cutting sutures or tissue.

Scissors should be held in the same way as artery forceps or needle holders.

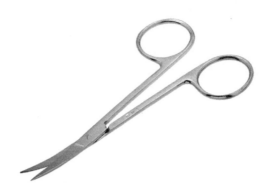

Figure 3.17 Curved sharp scissors.

Retractors

Retractors are used to keep tissues out of the way to improve the amount of access and visibility during operations. These can either be manual retractors that are used by the assistant to provide traction, or self-retaining retractors that use a mechanism to exert traction freeing up the assistant for other tasks.

When you first begin to assist in theatre, using retractors will be a common task that you will be able to help with. Knowing which retractor to use and how best to assist will prove invaluable for the operating surgeon and will demonstrate your understanding of surgical principles.

For retracting skin incisions, an excellent choice is the skin hook. This instrument can be used to manipulate the skin with the minimum of trauma.

Catspaw retractors, on the other hand, have a sharp 'claw' end that is used to hook skin edges without applying pressure to them. The other end of the retractor is a small, blunt, curved blade that can be used to gently move delicate tissues out of the operative field.

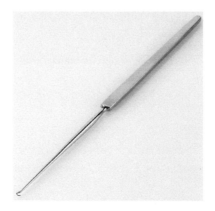

Figure 3.18 A skin hook.

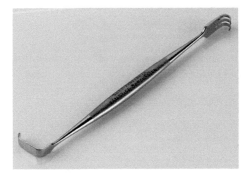

Figure 3.19 Catspaw retractor.

For deeper tissue retraction, longer retractors are crucial; Langenbeck retractors come in a variety of sizes and are commonly utilised.

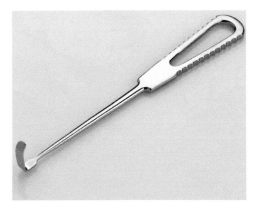

Figure 3.20 Langenbeck retractor.

Self-retractors come in different sizes and are used to retract at different depths. The Alms retractor is commonly used to retract superficial skin incisions. It operates with a screw thread to provide traction.

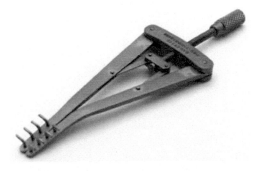

Figure 3.21 Alms self-retaining retractor.

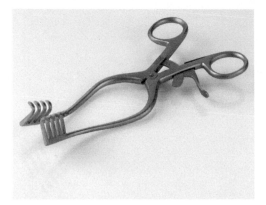

Figure 3.22 Travers self-retaining retractor.

For deeper operative fields, larger self-retaining retractors are used, such as Travers or Norfolk and Norwich self-retractors. These both use a ratchet mechanism to provide traction.

4 Sutures

Graeme M Downes

Classification of sutures

When thinking about sutures there are two things that need to be considered. The first is the suture itself – the material it is made from and its thickness. The second is the needle and what shape and size it is.

For the suture itself, the material can be categorised in three ways: absorbable or non-absorbable, braided or monofilament, natural or synthetic. All sutures fall into one of the options in each category. We will discuss these classifications before looking at some common suture materials at the end of this chapter to illustrate this categorisation.

Absorbable or non-absorbable

Sutures can be made from a material that is designed to retain its tensile strength indefinitely. These tend to be utilised either where there is a need for the strength to be maintained or a plan for removal later, and we use this for skin closure. Non-absorbable materials are also used where the strength must last indefinitely, such as vascular stents, tendon repairs or sternal wires. There is a second advantage with vascular or tendon repairs as the non-absorbable materials do not tend to be pro-inflammatory or pro-thrombotic so are used to ensure consistent outcomes.

Alternatively, sutures can be absorbable – these are materials with consistent and predictable rates of degradation that can be used where it is impractical or impossible to remove the sutures later. This may be for internal stitches, stiches in sensitive areas or in children, where removal would be uncomfortable for the patient.

DOI: 10.1201/b23298-4

Different types of absorbable sutures will break down at different rates, and for the common operations in your department, there will be a preference for certain types of sutures.

Monofilament or braided

The next consideration for your suture selection is the structure: this can be a single strand (a monofilament) or multiple strands (a braided suture).

Braided sutures tend to form more secure knots by virtue of the greater amount of friction they have, and also tend to be more effective at creating a seal. This makes then more useful for repairing bowel tissue, for example, but they are also commonly used for skin closure. The disadvantage is that the braided structure tends to create a capillary action, drawing fluid along the length of the suture, potentially increasing the risk of infection.

Monofilaments tend to be harder to tie and retain a degree of memory, i.e., a tendency to want to spring back to the shape it has been held in during storage. The lack of braided structure makes these sutures less likely to collect fluid and potentially reduces the risk of infection.

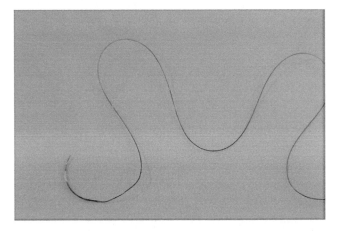

Figure 4.1 A good demonstration of the memory of monofilament sutures.

Natural or synthetic

This distinction has become less important over time; with the advent of many versatile synthetic materials the use of natural materials has diminished. The most utilised natural suture is silk, which is mainly used to secure drains.

Natural materials tend to have a greater risk of localised reactions, and because of their natural production don't have the same predictability of breakdown and strength over time that more homogenous synthetic materials do.

Some common sutures

Polyamide (nylon) sutures are **synthetic, non-absorbable, monofilament** sutures. Commonly these are used for skin closure where the intention is to remove the sutures in a defined amount of time.

Polyglactin sutures are **synthetic, absorbable, braided** sutures. Commonly used for deeper closures of structures, the more rapidly absorbed variation is often used for the closure of mucous membranes or nail beds.

Variations of **synthetic, absorbable, monofilament** sutures are manufactured – these tend to be combinations of different polymers. They are commonly used for intra dermal or sub dermal closure to bring larger wounds together.

Polydioxanone sutures (PDS) are also **synthetic, absorbable**, and **monofilament**. They have one of the longest retentions of strength times of all absorbable sutures and are used where consistent strength is needed, like fascial closures.

Suture size

Sutures come in a variety of diameters: the larger the diameter, the stronger the material, and it can provide greater tensile strength. The drawback is that the larger the suture size, the more destructive it is to the tissues and the greater the scarring. As a general rule, it is best to use the smallest diameter of suture that will provide enough tensile strength.

More strength is needed for a wound that will be subject to tension or highly mobile, such as extension surfaces of joints.

Sutures are sized from the largest, such as steel wire or some PDS being a size 2, moving to smaller size 1, and size 0 sutures, which are still some of the largest commonly used. Once sutures get smaller than this, they begin to be numbered 1-0, 2-0, 3-0 and so forth in decreasing size down to microsurgery sutures being 8-0 and smaller.

Needle selection

Needle selection is guided by the shape, size and cutting profile of the needle.

The needle shape can be straight or curved; curved needles are categorised by their length as well as their curvature, expressed as fractions of a complete circle. So, for example a 3/8 needle will be a 135° curve.

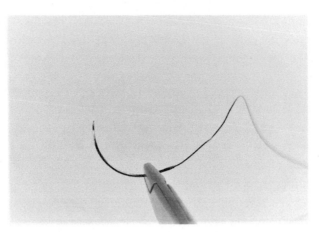

Figure 4.2 A 3/8 cutting needle.

The cutting profile of a needle can usually be described as 'cutting', where the cross section is a triangle with three sharp edges, or 'reverse cutting', also triangular in cross section but with a cutting surface on the outside of the needle curve. These needles have strong cutting properties and are used for passing through tough tissue, such as skin.

Tapered needles are circular in cross section with a pointed tip and are used for passing through tissue such as bowel or tendon with the minimal of trauma.

5 Tying surgical knots

Graeme M Downes

The knot should be tied as flat and small as possible to reduce its bulk. By utilising a secure technique, it will ensure the smallest secure knot possible.

The videos cited throughout this chapter can be viewed by scanning this QR code.

You should avoid crushing the suture material with the instruments as well as pulling on the suture excessively which risks snapping the material.

The tension of the knot should be enough to approximate the tissues without excessive tension that will impede healing.

Knots can be tied using instruments or by hand. Instrument ties will be more efficient with the suture material and are generally quicker to master but require more room for the movement of the instruments.

Instrument ties (Video 5.1)

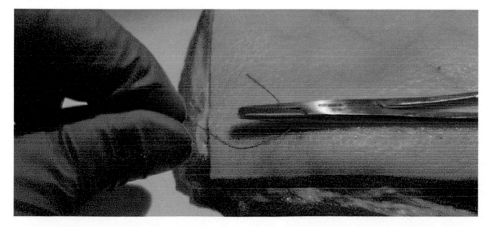

Figure 5.1 Starting position.

DOI: 10.1201/b23298-5

With the needle holders in your right hand, position them between the two ends of the suture with the long end with the needle nearest to you and the short end that is free furthest from you.

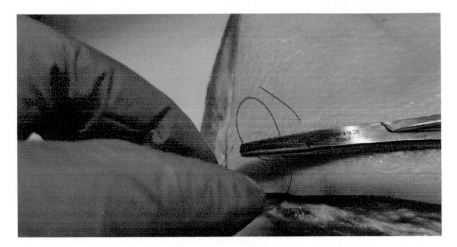

Figure 5.2 The first loop of the suture – do this twice.

Pick up the long end of the suture, being sure to do this away from the needle, and pass the suture around your needle holders **twice**.

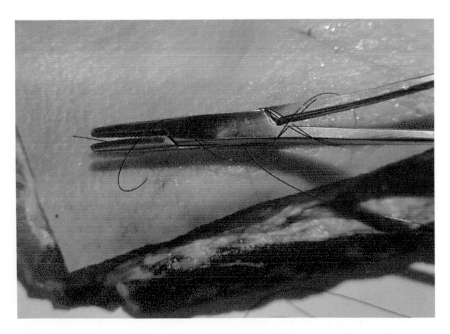

Figure 5.3 Pick up the short end with the needle holders.

Keeping the loops around the needle holders, use the instrument to pick up the short end.

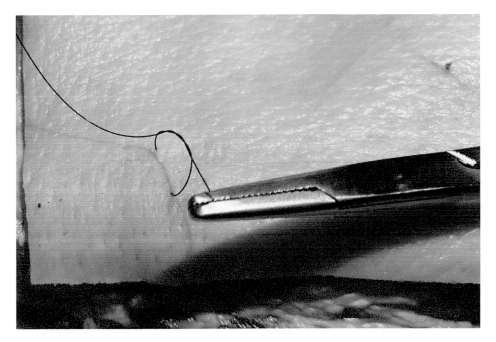

Figure 5.4 Creating the first knot.

Pull the short end towards you to lay your first flat knot.

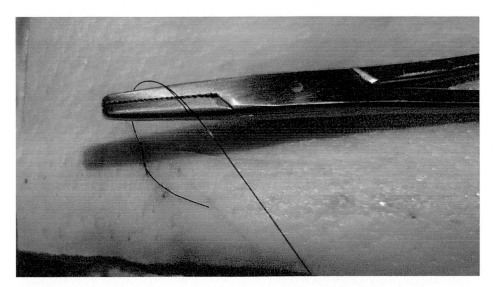

Figure 5.5 The starting position for the second throw.

Prepare for the second throw.

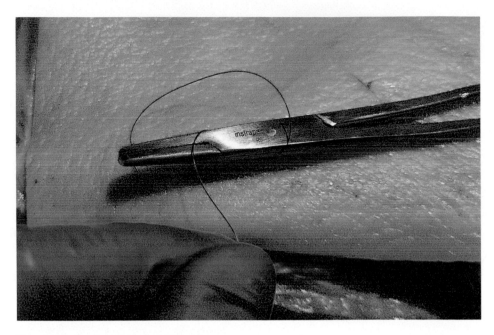

Figure 5.6 Starting the second throw.

Place your needle holders between the suture ends again, pick up the long end and pass **one** loop over the needle holders.

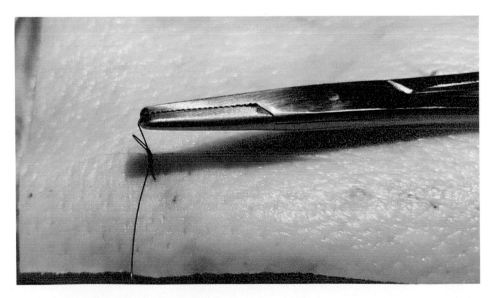

Figure 5.7 Completing the second throw.

Grasp the short end with the needle holders again and pull it away from you to make your second throw of the knot.

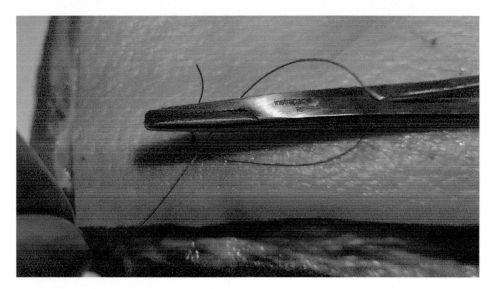

Figure 5.8 Starting the third throw.

Once more place your needle holders in the middle of the two suture ends and pass the long end around the instrument **once**.

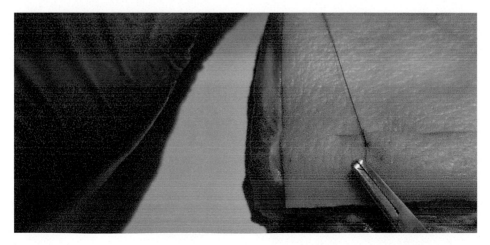

Figure 5.9 Completing the third throw.

Grasp the short end with the needle holders and pull the short end towards you to complete your square knot.

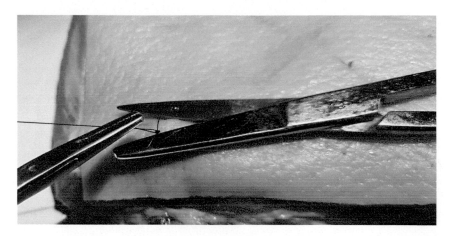

Figure 5.10 Cutting the suture ends.

If this was a real suture you would now cut the ends, leaving a good amount of excess in the case of a non-absorbable suture to make the eventual removal easier. You would trim an absorbable suture much closer.

Hand ties (Video 5.2)

With hand tying there are one-handed and two-handed techniques. Here we will work through a two-handed technique, the main principle being to alternate the direction you throw the knot. Throwing knots away from you and then towards you ensures that the knots lay flat and you create a correct surgeon's knot.

For this demonstration we will use a string with a white and a blue end for clarity.

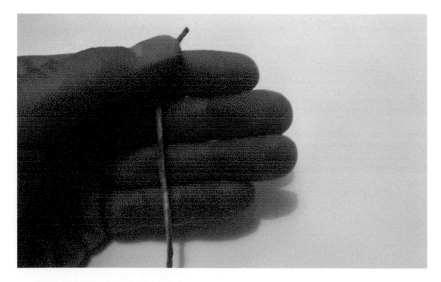

Figure 5.11 Placing the first suture end.

Start with the blue end running along the volar surface of your left fingers at the level of the proximal interphalangeal joints, with the cut end held on the index finger with the thumb.

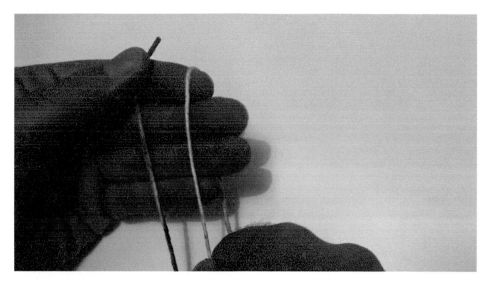

Figure 5.12 Placing the other suture end.

Bring the white end across your hand running from the index finger towards the little finger at the level of the distal interphalangeal joints, held with your right hand.

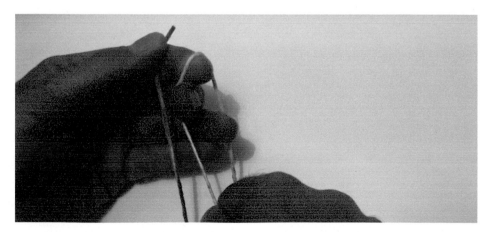

Figure 5.13 Starting your first throw.

Prepare for your first throw.

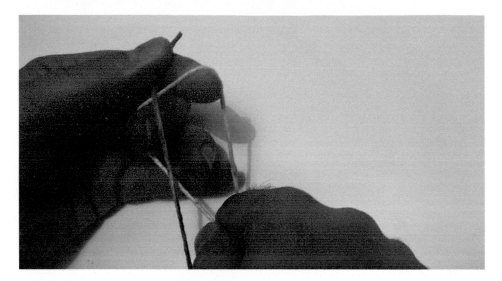

Figure 5.14 Bring your middle finger under the blue end.

Hook the distal phalanx of your middle finger on the white end and bring it under the blue end.

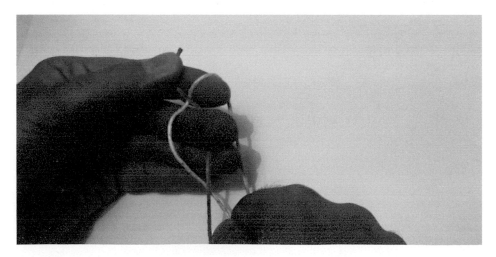

Figure 5.15 Grasp the blue end.

Extend the distal phalanx of your middle finger to grasp the blue end between your middle and ring fingers.

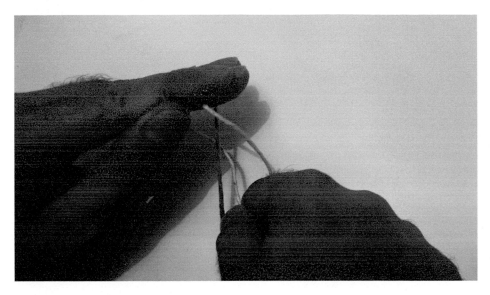

Figure 5.16 Pull the blue end through the loop.

Pronate your hand and pull the blue end through the loop you have created, releasing with your thumb at the same time.

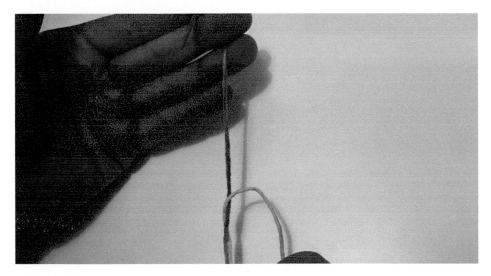

Figure 5.17 Pull the blue end to create your first knot.

Pull the blue end away from you to create the first flat knot.

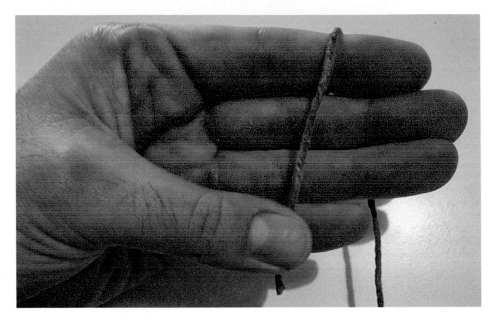

Figure 5.18 Starting the next throw.

By bringing your hand under the thread, the blue end will now be running down your hand ending at your little finger, where you should hold it with your thumb.

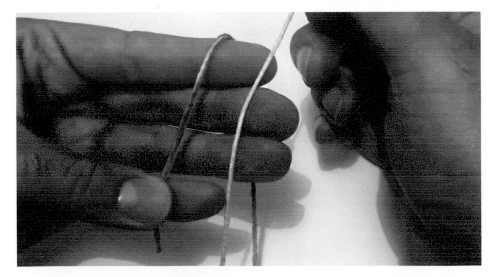

Figure 5.19 Position the white end of the string.

Run the white end along your palm towards your index finger.

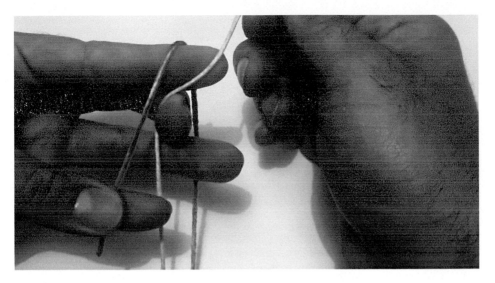

Figure 5.20 Bend your finger onto the thread as before.

Hook your middle finger on the white end as before.

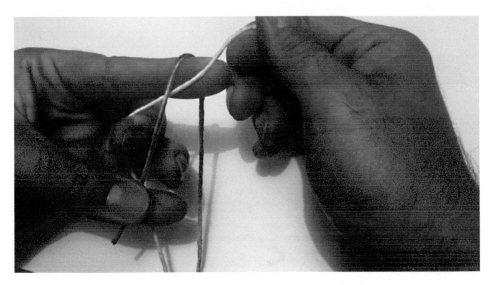

Figure 5.21 Hook your finger under the blue thread as before.

Repeat the same series of movements with the distal phalanx of your middle finger.

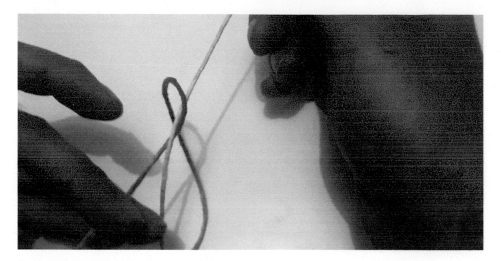

Figure 5.22 Now pull the blue thread **towards** you.

You should repeat these steps again to throw one more away from you and one more towards you.

This will create a double surgeons knot, which will be secure, but more throws can be added as needed.

When you have completed enough throws the suture ends can be cut.

Hand tying is a skill that requires practice to become fluent and does need to kept well practised. It is a useful skill for knot tying in confined spaces, such as tying off vessels or tying knots at depth, where instrument tying is not practical.

6 Local anaesthesia

Rituja Kamble

Local anaesthetic administration (Video 6.1)

The videos cited throughout this chapter can be viewed by scanning this QR code.

Prior to any basic surgical procedure, such as those outlined in this book, the area in question must be appropriately anaesthetised. Knowing how to safely dose and administer local anaesthetic is a crucial skill which will provide comfort for the patient and enable you to perform the procedure most effectively, optimising the outcome.

In this chapter you will learn about:

● Properties of local anaesthetics

● Safe dosing with and without adrenaline

● Infiltration technique

● Local anaesthetic toxicity

DOI: 10.1201/b23298-6

Properties of local anaesthetics

Local anaesthetic agents are membrane-stabilising compounds. In general, there are two classes of agent: amides and esters. The vast majority of agents we use in practice today are **amides**. Examples include lidocaine, bupivacaine, levobupivacaine, prilocaine. Esters have become less used in UK practice due to a higher risk of anaphylaxis related to secondary metabolites when compared to amides. Procaine is the only **ester** that is typically used in the UK today.

Local anaesthetic agents exert their action by interacting with **voltage-gated sodium channels** of sensory neurons to inhibit the influx of sodium ions across the cell membrane. This prevents formation of an action potential and therefore inhibits signal conduction and transmission. This renders the area in question insensitive to sharp, painful stimuli.

The onset of action and duration varies amongst local anaesthetic agents. When we compare the two commonly used agents, lidocaine and bupivacaine, we see that lidocaine has a **faster** onset of action but a **shorter** duration whereas bupivacaine has a **slower** onset of action but a **longer** duration. See Table 6.1 for more details.

Some formulations of local anaesthetic contain **adrenaline**, a potent vasoconstrictor which will reduce the rate of local anaesthetic absorption into the systemic circulation. This means the agent is effectively concentrated in the area for a longer period of time and enables the operator to potentially use a larger dose of local anaesthetic.

Adrenaline containing preparations

The use of adrenaline in local anaesthesia has several advantages. The vasoconstriction effect means that the local anaesthetic agent is concentrated in the area it has been infiltrated. This causes it to have a greater duration of action, and potentially enables the use of larger concentrations safely due to the slower systemic absorption.

The second effect is that the vasoconstriction reduces the amount of bleeding and can improve surgical visibility. It is important to note that this haemostatic effect is relatively slow to become effective so time should be allowed for this, should this be desired.

There is a commonly held view that adrenaline containing local anaesthetics should not be used in extremities such as the digits, penis or nose. The concern is that the vasoconstrictive effects of these preparations could lead to ischaemic damage. In the case of finger blocks, a Cochrane review found no evidence of any adverse effect.[1] With adrenaline being metabolised in 1–2 hours it is hard to explain why this would cause an ischaemic injury, when limb tourniquets are used frequently for a similar duration with no concerns. Be guided by local policy and your supervisors as to when it is appropriate to use an adrenaline containing local anaesthetic.

Be aware:

- Use adrenaline containing solutions in end arteriole territories with caution.

- Areas of localised infection (such as **an abscess**) will be more **acidic** than surrounding normal tissue. This may affect the action of the local anaesthetic and render it less effective.

- Avoid using these agents if the patient has a history of allergic reaction to local anaesthetic.

- Injecting local anaesthetic into a blood vessel or overdosing may lead to toxicity, which can be potentially dangerous for the patient. (Discussed later in this chapter).

- Local anaesthetics are metabolised by the liver and excreted through the urine so care should be taken with patients with renal or hepatic impairments.

- Adrenaline containing preparations should be used with caution in patients with ischaemic heart or peripheral disease. The vasoconstrictive effects could cause harm in these patients. If in doubt use a non-adrenaline preparation or seek specialist advice.

- Lidocaine is a cause of methemoglobinemia – if there is a past medical history of this then seek specialist advice.

Safe dosing of local anaesthetic

The most common agents used in clinical practice are **lidocaine, bupivacaine and levobupivacaine**. Prilocaine is also used on occasions.

Lidocaine

This can come in concentrations of 0.5%, 1% and 2% with or without adrenaline.

The maximum safe dosage of lidocaine in the product literature[2] is 4.5 mg/kg in adults and 3 mg/kg in children under 12. For the sake of simplicity and safety a default 3 mg/kg maximal dose is the safest practice. A maximum dose of 200 mg is recommended.

When using a 1% lidocaine with 1:200,000 adrenaline preparation the product literature[3] recommends a maximum of 7 mg/mL dose with a limit of 500 mg of lidocaine. This maximum dose of 500 mg is reached at just over 71 kg body weight.

There is a maximal dose of adrenaline that is safe for use, which is 4 micrograms/kg, or 200 micrograms maximum. When using any of the local anaesthetics with 1:200,000 adrenaline preparations described here, the maximum dose of the local anaesthetic will be reached first. The exceptions to this are the preparations of lidocaine with 1:80,000 adrenaline – with these the adrenaline is the limiting factor, giving a maximum dose of 16 mL.[4]

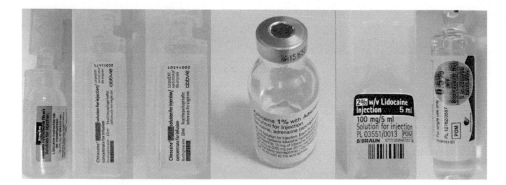

Figure 6.1 Some typical local anaesthetic agents.

Bupivacaine

This can come in concentrations of 0.25% and 0.5% with or without adrenaline.

Bupivacaine has the advantage of having a longer duration of effect – up to eight hours – but does also have a longer onset of action of between one and ten minutes.[5] Maximum recommended dosage is 2 mg/kg with a maximal dose of 150 mg.

Bupivacaine with adrenaline has the same maximal dose of 150 mg as plain bupivacaine and is generally recommended to be used up to 2 mg/kg. It has the advantage of longer duration of action over plain bupivacaine.

Levobupivacaine

Levobupivacaine is a chiral compound of bupivacaine and is intended to provide a greater duration of effect. The product literature concludes that it is equal in effectiveness to bupivacaine. It also has the same dosage considerations.[6]

The dose of local anaesthetic can increase if it is mixed with adrenaline. See Table 6.1 for the exact dosing.

Table 6.1 Maximum dose, onset of action and duration of commonly used local anaesthetic agents

Agent	Time of Onset	Time of Offset	Maximum Dose
Lidocaine	Within 2 minutes	Fast	3 mg/kg 200 mg max
Lidocaine with adrenaline	Within 2 minutes	Medium	7 mg/kg 500 mg max
Bupivacaine	Within 10 minutes	Medium	2 mg/kg 150 mg
Bupivacaine with adrenaline	Within 10 minutes	Long	2 mg/kg 150 mg
Levobupivacaine	Within 10 minutes	Medium	2 mg/kg 150 mg

Infiltration technique

The following will guide you in drawing up local anaesthetic and infiltrating it into tissues.

You will need:

1. Ampoule of local anaesthetic
2. 10 mL syringe
3. Drawing-up needle (ensure a filtered needle if you are using glass vials)
4. Injecting needle (ideally a blue or orange type)
5. Alcohol wipe
6. Gauze
7. Sharps bin

Check the expiry date of the local anaesthetic with a colleague and ensure it is within date.

Attach the drawing-up needle to the syringe, open the ampoule and aspirate its contents.

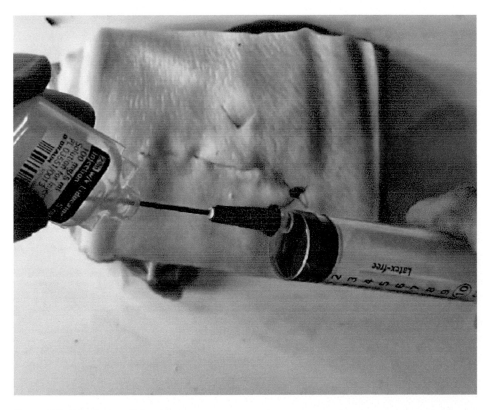

Figure 6.2 Drawing up lidocaine.

Remove the drawing-up needle from the syringe and dispose of it in the sharps bin. Replace the syringe with the injecting needle.

Prepare the target site with an alcohol wipe and insert the needle at a 30–45° angle into the skin. It should enter into the dermal plane. You should consider the anatomical course of the sensory nerves when starting your infiltration. Usually starting the block at the proximal side of the area will be the most effective.

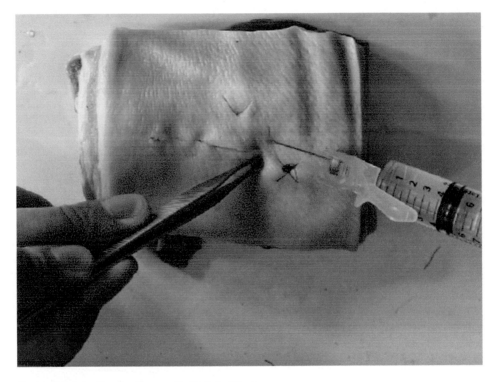

Figure 6.3 Injecting local anaesthetic into tissue.

Aspirate to ensure you have not entered a blood vessel.

Inject the local anaesthetic slowly into the tissue. Slow infiltration is more comfortable for the patient.

Injecting in a circle- or fan-like shape from a single entry point is also more comfortable for the patient. Another technique is to introduce the needle into the edges of a wound, again reducing the amount of skin trauma. Don't forget to aspirate each time before injecting. Use the gauze to dab the area clean of blood.

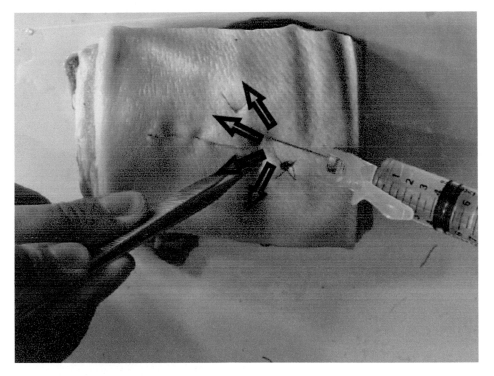

Figure 6.4 Injecting in a fan-like method.

If you have a skin lesion or cyst, infiltrate the tissue surrounding the lesion. This will render the target site painless. This is a **field block**.

When you have finished, dispose of the injecting needle in the sharps bin, dry the site and wash your hands. You can start to prepare for your surgical procedure while the anaesthetic takes effect. Test sharp sensation before starting your procedure.

Local anaesthetic toxicity

If an inappropriately large dose of local anaesthetic is administered or accidentally injected into a blood vessel, there is a risk of local anaesthetic toxicity. This can be potentially life-threatening, and care should be taken to identify the signs early and escalate it appropriately. The signs and symptoms of systemic toxicity can be subtle; they consist of **neurological** and **cardiovascular** sequelae which can occur immediately after IV injection or about 10–20 minutes after local infiltration.

Early signs and symptoms:

● Light-headedness

● Tinnitus

- Difficulty focusing vision
- Anxiety or agitation
- Drowsiness or disorientation
- Confusion
- Metallic taste
- Perioral or tongue numbness

Cardiovascular signs and symptoms:

- Bradycardia
- Hypotension
- Dysrhythmias
- Cardiovascular collapse
- Asystole

Neurological signs and symptoms:

- Seizures
- Slurred speech
- Coma

There may be other symptoms present such as respiratory depression and apnoea.

Immediate actions:

1. Stop the procedure and cease administration of the local anaesthetic immediately
2. Call for help
3. Ensure the patient's airway is maintained and administer high-flow oxygen
4. Obtain IV access and perform an ECG
5. Administer antidote if available (Intralipid)

Further management will be directed by the patient's symptoms. More information can be found in the Appendix.

Notes

1   Prabhakar, H., Rath, S., Kalaivani, M., and Bhanderi, N., 2015. Adrenaline with lidocaine for digital nerve blocks. *Cochrane Database of Systematic Reviews*, 2020(11).

2 The electronic medicines compendium, 2022. Lidocaine Hydrochloride Injection BP 1% w/v - Summary of Product Characteristics (SmPC) - (emc). [online] Available at: https://www.medicines.org.uk/emc/product/6277/smpc

3 The electronic medicines compendium, 2022. Xylocaine 1% with Adrenaline - Summary of Product Characteristics (SmPC) - (emc). [online] Available at: https://www.medicines.org.uk/emc/product/2397/smpc

4 Septodont, 2022. Summary of Product Characteristics - Lignospan special. [online] Septodont.co.uk. Available at: https://www.septodont.co.uk/sites/uk/files/2020-11/LIGNOSPAN-UK_SmPC_APP_en_201807.pdf].

5 The electronic medicines compendium. 2022. Bupivacaine 0.5%w/v solution for injection - Summary of Product Characteristics (SmPC) - (emc). [online] Available at: https://www.medicines.org.uk/emc/medicine/29727#gref

6 The electronic medicines compendium, 2022. Chirocaine 2.5 mg/mL solution for injection/concentrate for solution for infusion - Summary of Product Characteristics (SmPC) - (emc). [online] Medicines.org.uk. Available at: https://www.medicines.org.uk/emc/product/1555/smpc#PHARMACODYNAMIC_PROPS

7 Suture techniques

Graeme M Downes

Wound healing

Wound healing occurs in four stages[1]:

- Haemostasis
- Inflammation

The videos cited throughout this chapter can be viewed by scanning this QR code.

DOI: 10.1201/b23298-7

- Proliferation
- Remodelling

Haemostasis

Vasoconstriction of injured vessels occurs on injury, after which platelets are activated to form a platelet-fibrin plug, which produces growth factors to promote wound healing.

Inflammation: Days 1–6

After the formation of the initial clot, vasodilatory signals – such as histamine, serotonin and nitric oxide – reverse the vasoconstriction and allows for increased blood flow to the wound. Platelet signalling molecules promote the coagulation cascade and the innate immune system. Cell signalling molecules are released that cause the migration of neutrophils and macrophages to the wound. These cells carry out phagocytosis of debris and dead cellular components. This migration of immune cells is facilitated by these vasodilatory compounds and is why there is a degree of erythema and swelling during the wound healing process. It is the macrophages that are most critical for wound healing as they are the major cellular component until the proliferation of fibroblasts.

Proliferative phase: Day 4 – Week 3

These immune cells begin to release vascular endothelial growth factor (VEG-F), PDGF-B and initial extracellular matrix, promoting the formation of new blood vessels and granulation tissue; further angiogenesis is stimulated by a low oxygen environment and higher lactate concentration.

As collagen begins to replace the initial extracellular matrix, there is a migration of myofibroblasts that utilise actin and myosin to begin to contract the wound and aid natural closure. Epithelisation begins to occur at this stage.

Remodelling: One year or longer

The final stage is then the gradual remodelling of collagen within the wound to form a mature scar, a process that can take over a year to fully complete.

Factors affecting wound healing

There are factors which will delay the process of wound healing; broadly these will be patient factors and surgical factors (which will be discussed later).

The first stage which can be affected by patient factors is the inflammation stage: it may be that there is poor blood flow to the wound area, as in vascular disease, renal failure or a distal or poorly supplied area of the body. Smoking is a significant risk to wound healing due to its vasoconstrictive effects and carbon monoxide binding preferentially to haemoglobin. There is also Hydrogen Cyanide in cigarette smoke that acts as a direct respiratory poison. Conversely, increased delivery of oxygen to wounded tissue has been found to aid wound healing: this is the basis of hyperbaric oxygen therapy.

It may be that there is immunosuppression that impedes the activity of the leukocytes, such as corticosteroid use, immune modulating drugs, malnutrition, advanced age, AIDS or diabetes mellitus.

The inflammatory response may be exaggerated or abnormal, such as in infected wounds. This can lead to chronic inflammation and chronic non-healing wounds.

The proliferation stage can be abnormal, resulting in excessive granulation tissue. This can lead to granuloma formation if left untreated. Radiation therapy leads to DNA damage and a reduction in epithelisation, and increased rates of dehiscence.

The aim of wound management is to ensure that the right treatment is carried out to allow for the quickest wound healing with the least morbidity. Broadly speaking this will be wound cleaning and debridement of dead tissue where necessary, reducing the inflammatory stimulus, and wound closure to minimise the amount of proliferation and remodelling that is required.

Wound cleaning

Wounds should always be cleaned – even if they appear to be clean there can be debris that is not visible in the wound that will delay the healing process and risk infection.

If the mechanism of injury suggests a foreign body within the wound – such as a laceration with wood/thorns or other organic material, broken glass or high-energy gravel injuries – then exploration and, if appropriate, imaging should be carried out. We will discuss wound debridement and cleaning in a later chapter. In this case we are considering a visibly clean wound. The wound should be irrigated with 0.9% saline: the amount of irrigation will depend on the case, but a generous amount – such as 500 mL to 1 litre – is usually appropriate.

If there are concerns over contamination of the wound, then a cleaning solution, such as povidone iodine, can be used. In these cases, it is usually inappropriate to immediately close the wound and a delayed closure strategy is advised.

How best to manage a wound?

As a general principle, the approach to managing a wound should be the least invasive method that will achieve good tissue coverage, attaining a good result for form and function.

With this idea in mind there is a 'Reconstructive Ladder' that should be kept in mind. The simpler techniques at the bottom of the ladder are less likely to have complications and should be utilised where they will have a good functional and cosmetic outcome:

- Free flap

- Distant pedicle flap

- Local flap

- Full thickness skin grafts

- Split thickness skin grafts

- Delayed primary closure

- Direct closure

- Secondary intention closure

Putting the ladder into practice, if there is a laceration that has just penetrated the superficial dermis (a papercut for example), then allowing that to heal by secondary intention is appropriate. Attempting to suture such a wound would involve more iatrogenic harm than the wound itself.

A wound that is full thickness through the dermis may well be best managed with direct closure and the way we approach this is down to a combination of patient preference, appropriate selection of technique and the skill and experience of the clinician.

The first consideration should be if the wound can be allowed to heal by secondary intention, potentially supported by adhesive wound closure strips. Would this provide enough strength to prevent the wound opening during day-to-day movements? Can the wound be brought together with good closure to prevent wound healing and an excessive scar?

Wound closure glue can be a good option: it can usually be used without needing local anaesthesia and is a quick technique. Some considerations here are that the glue is not particularly strong and is very difficult to use in large wounds, so should only be considered for small wounds that are not likely to experience much tension. It should also be noted that clinician skill has a large role with wound glue: the glue itself forms an inert plug and should not be used to fill a wound, as this will lead to a wide scar. The glue should instead be applied to a wound after the edges have been brought together in good approximation.

Suture decision making

As discussed earlier, you should aim to choose the smallest diameter of suture that will provide enough tensile strength. In practical terms, a 4-0 suture is usually appropriate for a limb, with a larger 3-0 for the trunk or back, or a smaller 5-0 (or even smaller) for the hands or face. These are not universal rules and adaption will be necessary depending on patient or surgical factors.

When deciding on where in the wound to place your sutures, you should be aiming to accomplish a good wound closure with the minimum number of sutures. A good method for doing this when you first start is to divide the wound in two and place your first suture there. If there are further sutures needed, these can then be placed halfway between each wound end and the midpoint. With larger wounds you can keep dividing the remaining wound in half to place further sutures.

In the upcoming sections you will learn several suture techniques. As you become more practised, you will learn which techniques are best suited to the size of the wound, the skin quality and the tension required.

Simple interrupted (Video 7.1)

A technique characterised by singular sutures that are inserted and tied separately, useful for closing simple wounds. You should become confident with this technique before moving on to the more complex techniques later in this chapter.

Start by using your toothed forceps to gently expose the wound edge furthest from you.

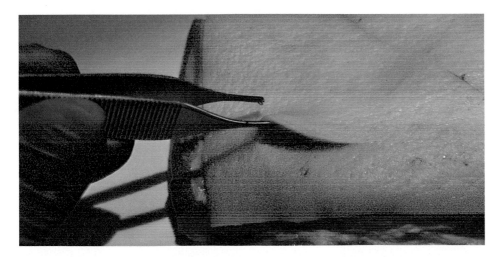

Figure 7.1 Lift the wound edge.

We are using toothed forceps to minimise the damage to the skin edges. With time you should aim to manipulate the skin with the minimum of gripping, relying more on the tooth of the forceps to lift the skin. You should now be able to confirm that there are no nerves, vessels or other structures that could be damaged by your intended suture placement.

With the skin edge lifted you should press the needle into the skin perpendicularly, then with a rotation of the wrist (supination in this case), move the needle through the skin.

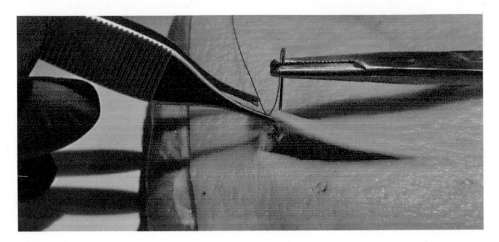

Figure 7.2 Pass the needle into the skin edge.

Once the needle has been passed through the skin, it can be grasped with the forceps and moved out of the wound.

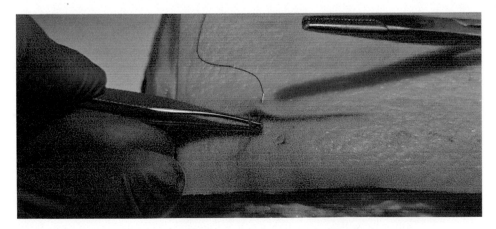

Figure 7.3 Draw the needle through the wound edge.

The suture can now be drawn through to leave just enough material on the short end to knot on to.

Now the skin edge nearest you is lifted with the forceps in the same way as before, once more ensuring that there are no structures at risk of damage.

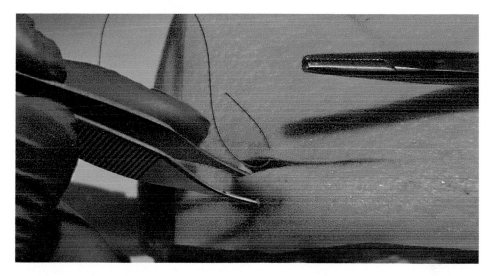

Figure 7.4 Draw the suture material through and then lift the nearest side of the wound.

The needle is now passed through the skin edge nearest you, but this time from the deep surface out to the superficial side. Pass the needle through the skin using a supination action, before grasping with the forceps to pull excess suture material through.

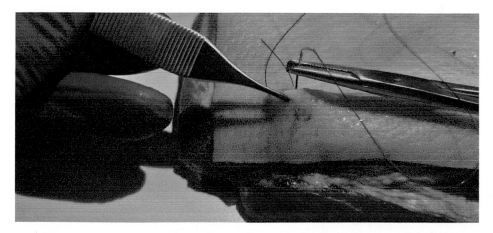

Figure 7.5 Draw the needle through the wound edge.

It is important to ensure that the suture passes between points on the two skin edges that are in line with each other and are the same distance from the wound edges. If there is a discrepancy, then there will be problems with the closure.

Now your first suture can be tied as discussed in Chapter 5.

The needle holders should be placed between the two ends of the suture as pictured.

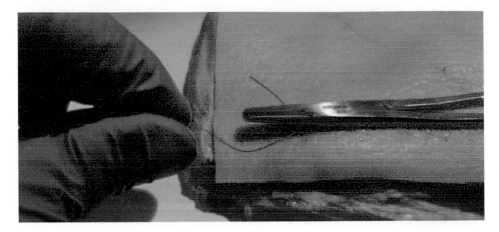

Figure 7.6 Start with your needle holders between the two suture ends.

Loop the suture **twice** around the needle holders.

You should take care to hold the suture material away from the needle to avoid injury. The short end can then be picked up in the needle holders and pulled towards you. This swapping of the suture ends is vital to lay down flat and secure knots.

Place the needle holders between the two ends of the suture and loop the long end around the instrument **once** before pulling the short end **away** from you.

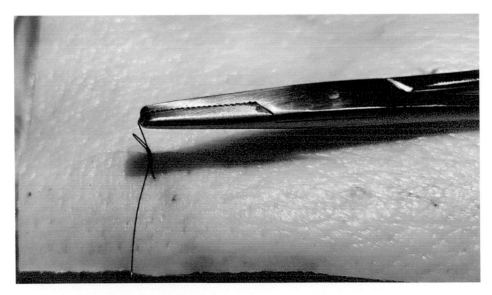

Figure 7.7 The second throw of the knot.

This completes the second throw of your knot.

For the final knot, place your needle holders between the ends of the sutures and loop the long end around the instrument **once**. Grasp the short end of the suture with the needle holders. Then pull that short end **towards** you, completing the third throw of your knot.

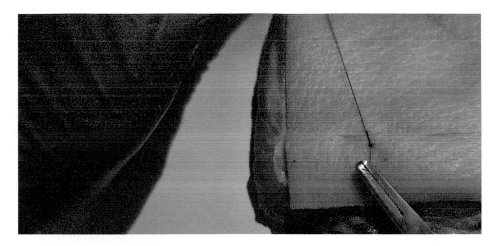

Figure 7.8 The third throw of the knot.

Cut the ends of your suture: this completes your first suture. You can now repeat this process to close the whole wound.

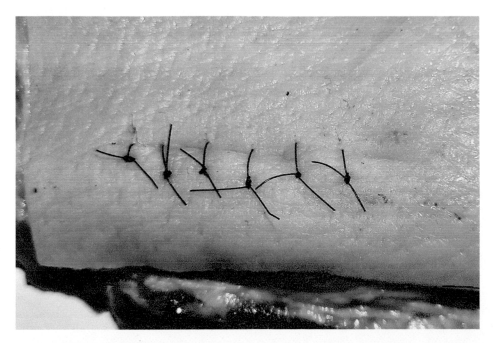

Figure 7.9 The completed wound closure.

Once you have mastered the simple interrupted suture you can move on to practising more complex types. The simple interrupted suture will always be a mainstay of your skills, but the following techniques will prove to be useful tools you can draw on to achieve a good closure for a variety of wounds.

Horizontal mattress (Video 7.2)

The horizontal mattress suture is useful for closing skin under tension or that is particularly fragile. This technique uses two passes of the material which spreads the tension and moves it away from the wound edges. It also everts the skin edges which, as the wound heals and there is a degree of contraction, helps with a better cosmetic appearance.

The start is the same as the simple interrupted suture: you should pass the suture through both edges of the wound.

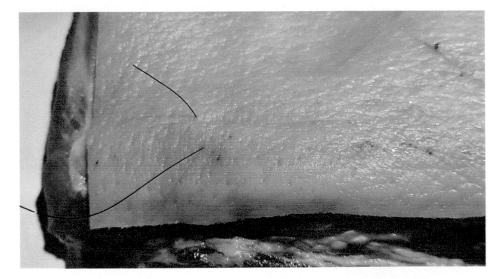

Figure 7.10 The first step is to carry out the start of an interrupted suture.

Once you have done this, instead of tying this suture as you would a simple interrupted one, you should pass the suture back through both edges of the wound.

To do this you should reverse the needle in the needle holders so that the point faces away from you. Using a backhand technique – that is pronation of the instrument – you can pass the suture back through the wound edges.

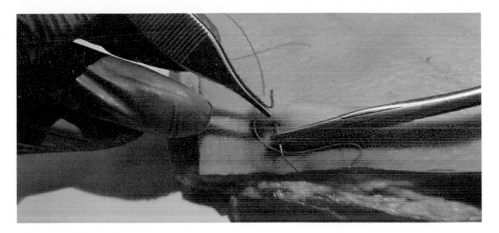

Figure 7.11 Pass the needle back through the wound, backhand.

The final suture should look like the image below: the four points at which the suture passes through the skin should be uniform in distance and depth, forming as close to right angles as possible between the four points.

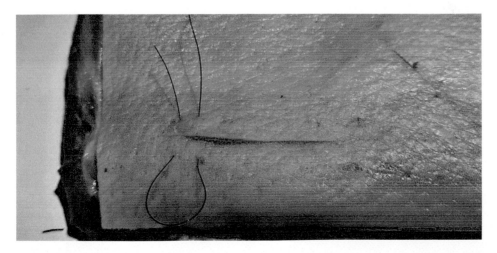

Figure 7.12 The completed suture before tying.

The knot can then be tied in the same way as before and the suture trimmed. Note the eversion of the skin edges.

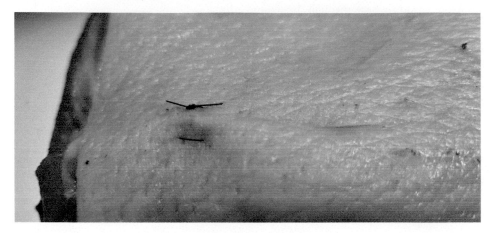

Figure 7.13 Complete your suture by tying and cutting the ends.

Vertical mattress (Video 7.3)

The vertical mattress suture has the same advantages as the horizontal mattress but can be used to distribute skin tension further from the skin edges and so can be more appropriate for fragile skin.

The first pass should be the same as the interrupted suture.

As with the horizontal suture, you should then reverse mount the needle.

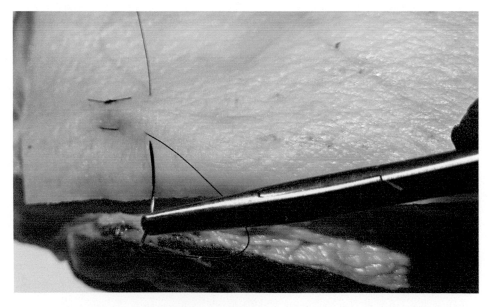

Figure 7.14 Start your vertical mattress by taking your first bite then backhand mount your needle.

Now pass the needle back through the wound edges, but this time through two points nearer the wound edges, and shallower than the first pass – ideally mid dermal rather than full thickness.

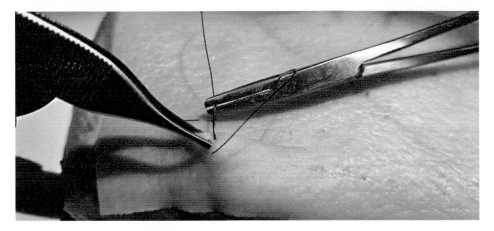

Figure 7.15 Now pass your needle back through, closer to the wound edges than before.

The final suture should follow this pattern.

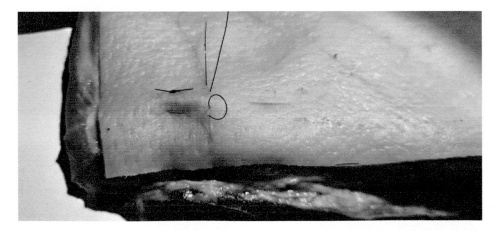

Figure 7.16 The completed vertical mattress suture before tying.

The suture can then be tied and trimmed, everting the skin edges and creating a good wound closure.

Here you can see both the horizontal and vertical mattress sutures.

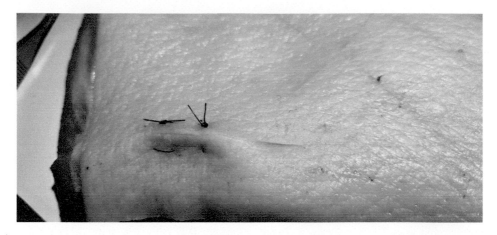

Figure 7.17 Now tie the suture to complete it.

Corner stitch (Video 7.4)

A type of stitch that is used to close corners of wounds with less risk of trauma to the narrow skin bridge. This minimises the risk of causing avascular necrosis at the apex of the corner.

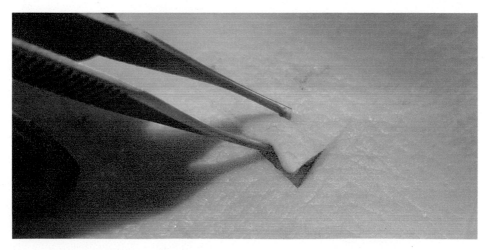

Figure 7.18 A typical corner flap.

First pass the suture through one of the skin edges facing the corner. This is the same starting movement as the interrupted suture.

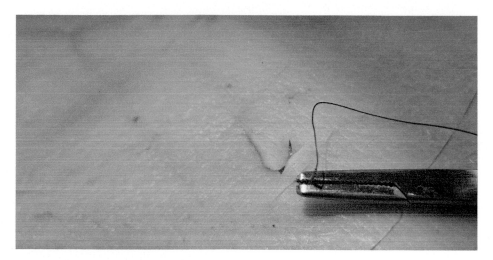

Figure 7.19 The starting movement.

Draw the suture through the skin edge.

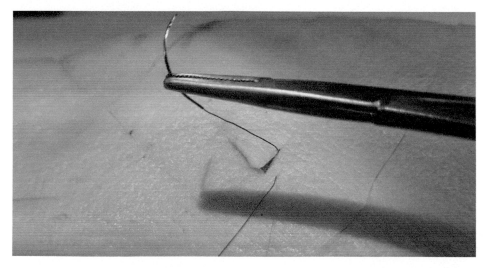

Figure 7.20 Completing the first pass of the suture.

Now pass the suture through the dermis of the skin corner, avoiding breeching the epithelium.

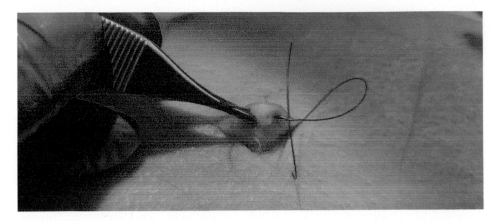

Figure 7.21 Pass the needle along the dermal layer.

Then pass the suture through the other skin edge facing the corner, at the same depth and mirror position to where you started.

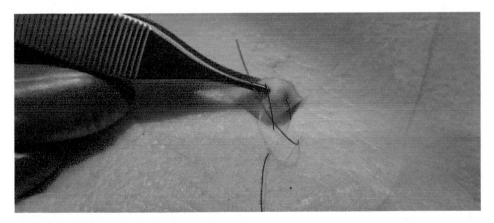

Figure 7.22 The last pass of the suture.

Tie the ends of the suture and cut. You should have a suture that is mainly sub epithelial.

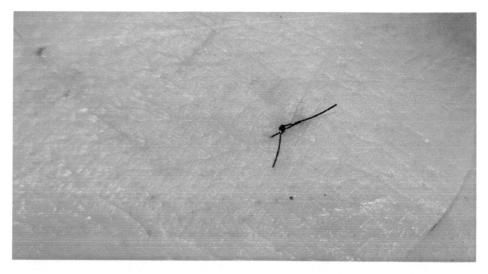

Figure 7.23 The completed suture.

Deep dermal (Video 7.5)

A type of stitch that is used to close deeper wounds with less risk of dehiscence and excess tension. An absorbable suture is used.

Pass the needle through the deep dermis of the wound edge nearest you – this should be from the deepest point to the more superficial dermis. Make sure you do not go into the epidermis.

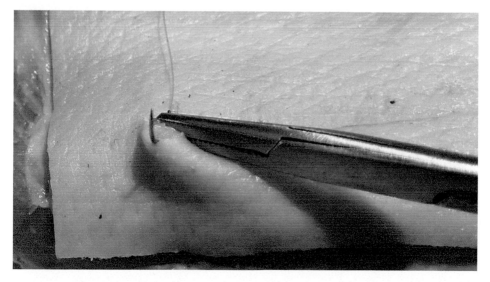

Figure 7.24 The first dermal bite.

Pull the suture through then pronate your hand to pass the needle through the dermis on the far side of the wound. This should be from the more superficial dermis to the deep dermis.

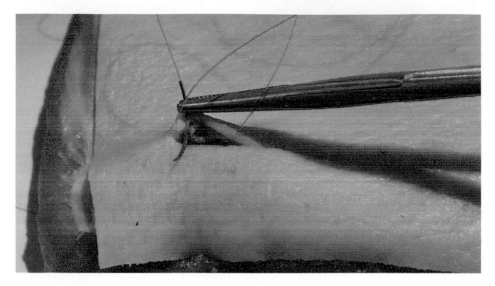

Figure 7.25 The second dermal bite.

Now knot the suture using a standard surgical knot. Ensure that you tighten the knot in line with the wound to ensure the knot is buried.

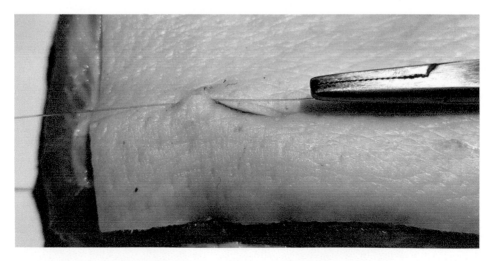

Figure 7.26 Tying the stitch.

Once the knot is tightened, cut the suture ends flush with the skin.

Subcuticular (Video 7.6)

A type of stitch that is used to close skin edges with the whole suture being below the epidermis. An absorbable monofilament should be used.

In the video accompanying this section, a dyed nylon suture has been used to enable better visibility.

First carry out a deep dermal suture like we saw in the last section. For the ease of using your needle holders in your right hand, start at the most right-hand edge of the wound. This will allow the subcuticular stitch to be carried out with the more ergonomic forehand movement.

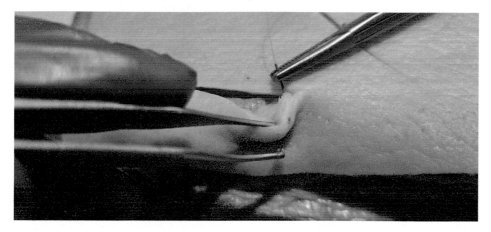

Figure 7.27 Starting the first stitch of the subcuticular.

You can see that we have once again passed the needle from the deep to superficial dermis on the near side of the wound and then from the superficial to the deep dermis on the far side of the wound.

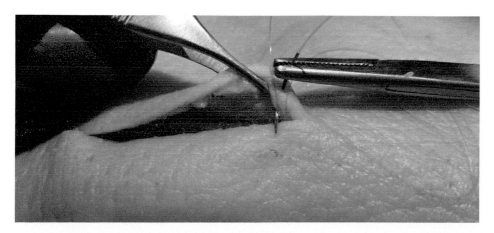

Figure 7.28 Taking the second bite for the initial stitch.

Once you have completed the first dermal suture, cut the short end of the suture flush with the skin.

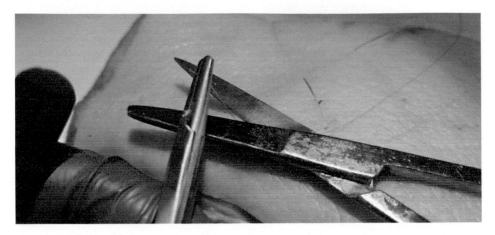

Figure 7.29 Cut only the short end of the suture.

Now pass the needle along the dermis at the wound edge, avoiding the epidermis.

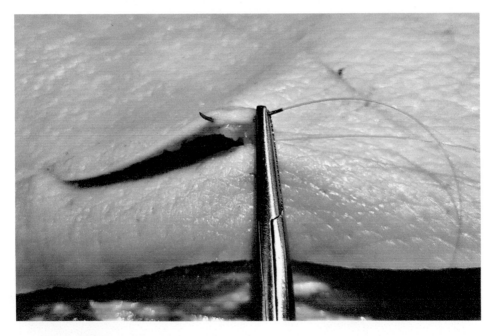

Figure 7.30 Take a superficial parallel bite.

Then pass the needle though the dermis on the near wound edge, starting slightly to the right of the point at which your first bite finished. Again, be sure to place the needle only in the superficial dermis.

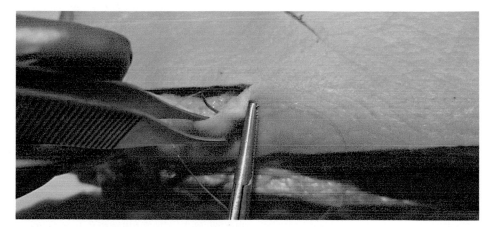

Figure 7.31 Take the next superficial dermal bite on the other side of the wound.

Continue to pass the suture through the dermis on each side of the wound.

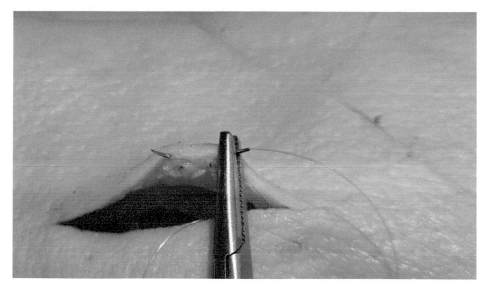

Figure 7.32 Continue this process along the length of the wound.

Continue to take subcuticular bites until you have closed the wound edges and do not pull through your last stich.

We will now complete this suture with an Aberdeen knot.

Start by putting your index and thumb through the loop created by your last bite.

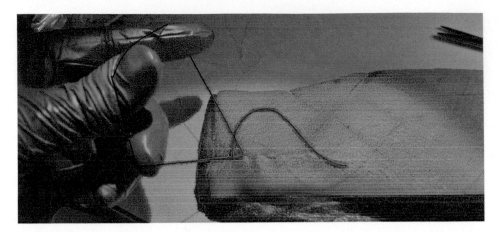

Figure 7.33 Starting the Aberdeen knot – the suture has been highlighted for ease of visibility.

Pinch the long piece of suture with the needle on.

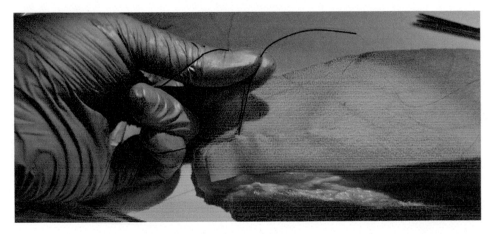

Figure 7.34 Pinch the end of the suture with the needle on.

Pull it through the loop, creating another loop. Tighten the first loop by pulling on the lower limb of your new loop.

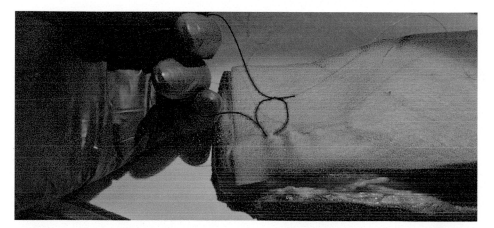

Figure 7.35 Pull that piece of suture through to create a new loop.

Once you have done this three times, pass the long end of the suture through your loop.

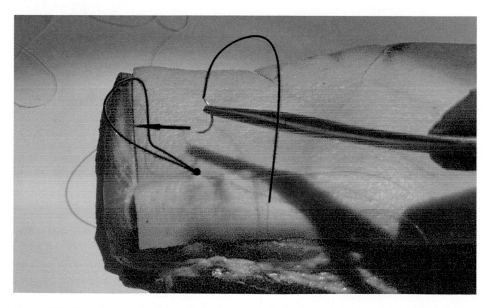

Figure 7.36 Pass the needle through the loop to lock the knot.

Pull to tighten and lock.

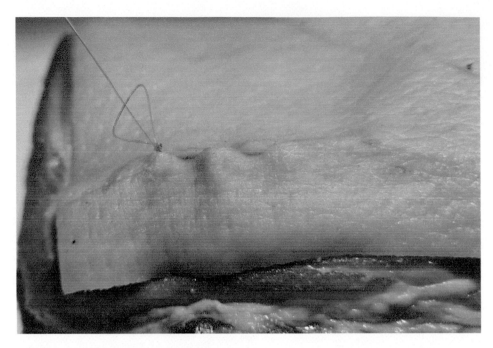

Figure 7.37 Pull the needle to tighten the knot.

Pass the needle into the wound line and out to the skin at the apex.

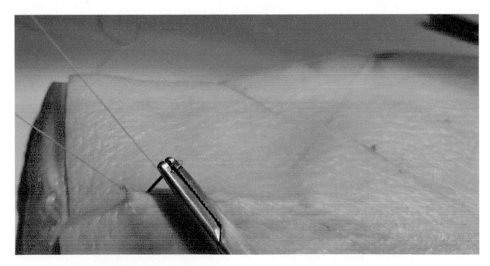

Figure 7.38 Burying the knot.

Prepare to bury the knot.

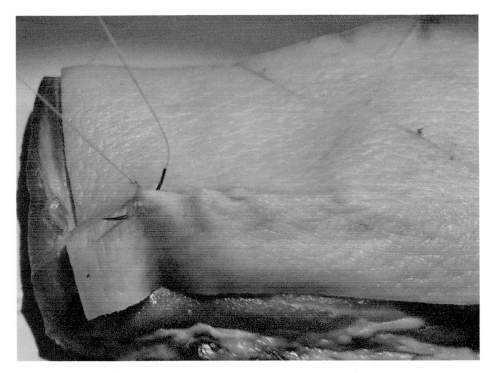

Figure 7.39 Pass the needle out at the apex of the wound.

Pull this tight to bury the knot within the wound and cut the end of the suture flush with the skin.

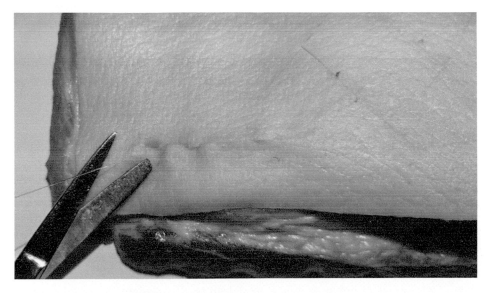

Figure 7.40 Cut the suture flush with the skin.

Locking techniques

There is a variation of the horizontal mattress where the long end of the suture is passed through a loop to create a locking knot that is less prone to coming loose during knotting. This is particularly useful for wounds under tension.

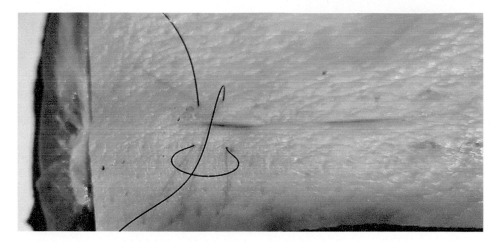

Figure 7.41 A type of locking suture.

Tendon repair

When it comes to repairing a flexor tendon, there are various techniques that are used to create the core repair, holding the tendon in position. There are also various techniques for carrying out an epitendonous repair after the core repair.

The principle of repairing any tendon is to create a strong repair without too much bulk, such that the repair glides freely and does not become obstructed.

A monofilament is used for these repairs to avoid sawing the tendon with a braided suture. Either a non-absorbable suture, or a suture with a very long absorption time such as PDS, is used. This ensures a long-lasting repair that maintains its tensile strength long enough for the tendon to heal.

In this section we will cover two core repair techniques – the modified Kessler and the Adelaide repair – as well as a continuous technique for epitendonous repair.

Modified Kessler technique

This is a more straightforward repair that bridges the site of injury with two strands of suture. It is a quick technique and more feasible in smaller tendons.

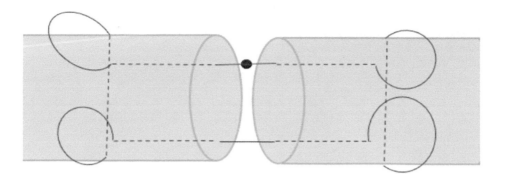

Figure 7.42 A schematic of a completed modified Kessler tendon repair.

In all tendon repairs it is important to minimise the handling of the tendon and you should aim to grasp the tendon only on the epitendonous sheath with non-toothed forceps to avoid fraying the core of the tendon.

In a real case you may need to trim the tendon ends to create a better surface to oppose during the repair, and you may find it necessary to anchor the tendons in place. You should seek advice on this depending on the specific case.

First identify the cut ends of the tendon and ensure that they align.

Grasp the epitendonous layer of the tendon with your non-toothed forceps.

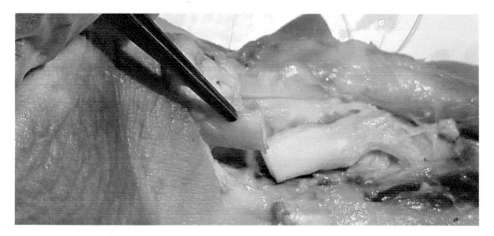

Figure 7.43 Grasping the tendon.

Pass the needle into the tendon end, parallel to the tendon. You should aim to pass it along the centre of the tendon.

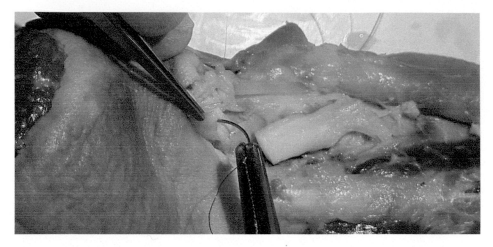

Figure 7.44 Passing the needle into the tendon.

Aim to emerge on the superficial side of the tendon around 1 cm away from the cut end.

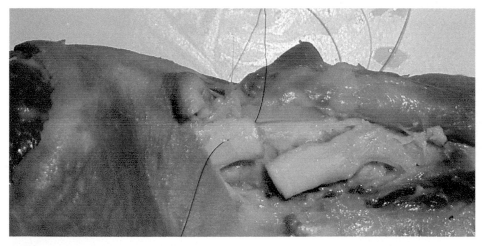

Figure 7.45 The first pass of the suture.

Now pass the suture perpendicular to the tendon to come out on the other side. Note that the free end of the suture is held with a clip to prevent it slipping.

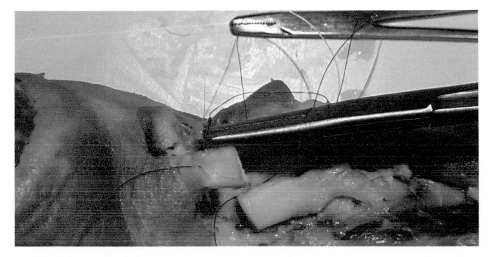

Figure 7.46 Pass the needle through the side of the tendon.

Note that as you pull the suture through it creates this loop that helps to anchor the repair in the tendon.

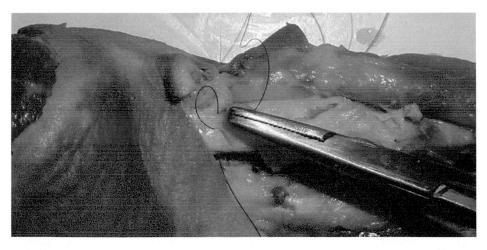

Figure 7.47 This creates a loop anchor in the tendon.

Now pass the needle back along the tendon towards the cut end, mirroring the first pass.

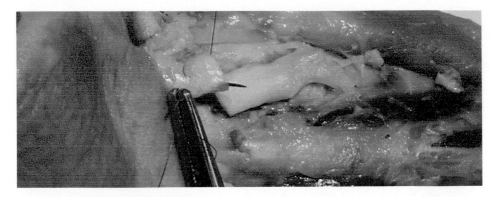

Figure 7.48 Pass the needle back through the tendon.

This creates another loop of suture to grasp the tendon.

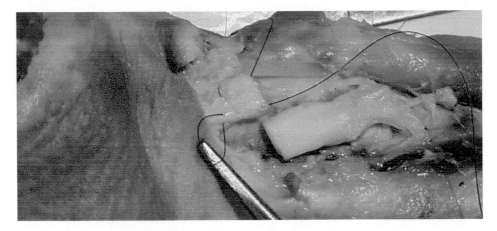

Figure 7.49 This creates a second loop anchor in the tendon.

Now pass the needle down the length of the other cut end, aiming to come out on the superficial side around 1 cm away from the cut end.

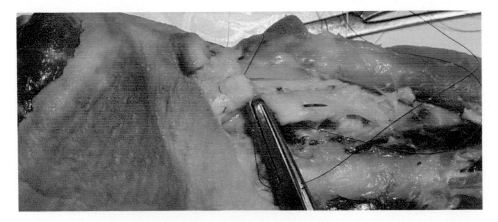

Figure 7.50 Pass the needle through the other end of the tendon.

In a similar way to the other side of the repair, now pass the needle perpendicularly across the tendon.

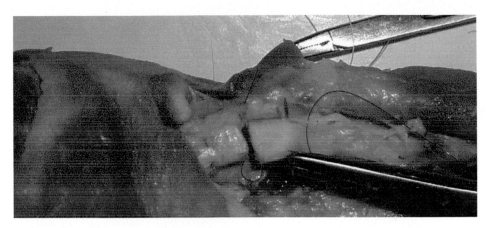

Figure 7.51 Pass the needle through the side of the tendon.

Once again this creates another loop.
Now pass the needle along the length of the tendon towards the cut end.

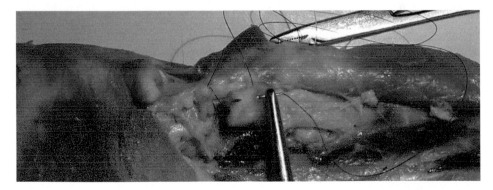

Figure 7.52 Pass the needle back through the tendon.

This creates a fourth loop anchor in the tendon.
Now take the clip off the loose end of the suture and tie a surgeon's knot, ensuring it is buried within the repair.

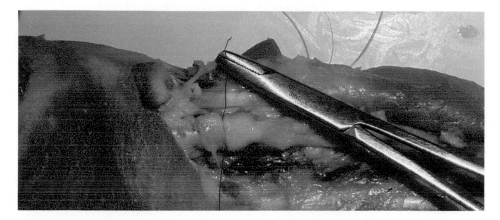

Figure 7.53 Tie your repair.

Cutting the suture ends should result in a completely buried knot.

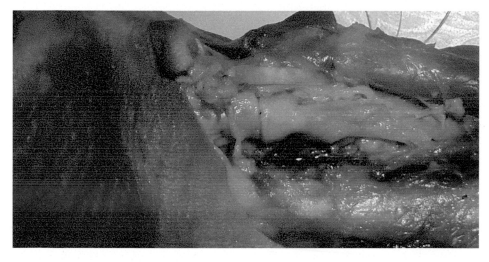

Figure 7.54 Your completed tendon repair.

The ends of your tendon repair should be opposed with no gapping, but not so tight that there is any compression.

Adelaide repair

The Adelaide repair utilises four strands between the cut tendon ends. This results in a more robust repair but can be difficult to achieve in smaller tendons.

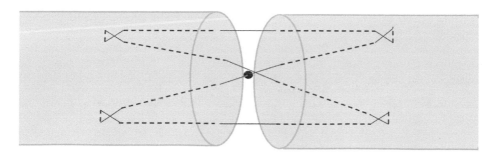

Figure 7.55 A schematic of a completed Adelaide tendon repair.

Starting in the middle, pass the needle along the tendon aiming to come out 1 cm along the cut end but close to the near side of the tendon.

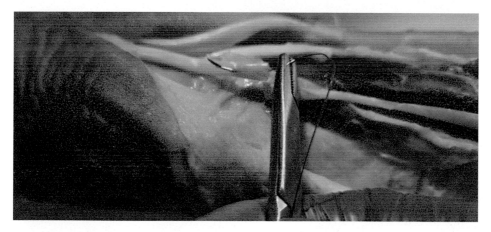

Figure 7.56 Your first bite of the tendon.

After this lengthwise bite, take a small perpendicular bite moving away from you.

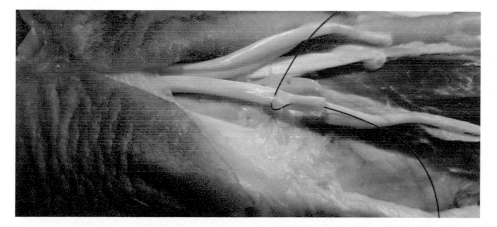

Figure 7.57 Your first anchoring bite of the tendon.

Now pass the needle along the tendon parallel to it and emerge on the cut end close to the edge nearest you.

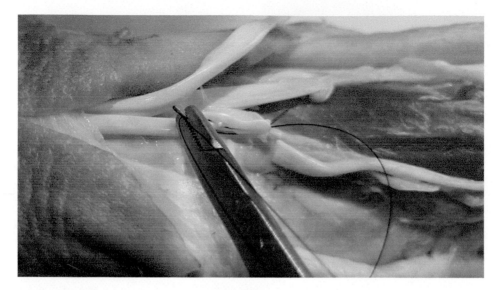

Figure 7.58 Pass the needle back down the tendon.

This should result in two strands that are anchored to the cut tendon.

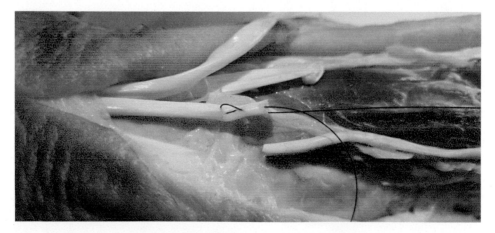

Figure 7.59 The first stage of the repair.

Now pass the needle down the other cut tendon end, aiming to be parallel to the edge and emerging 1 cm along the superior side.

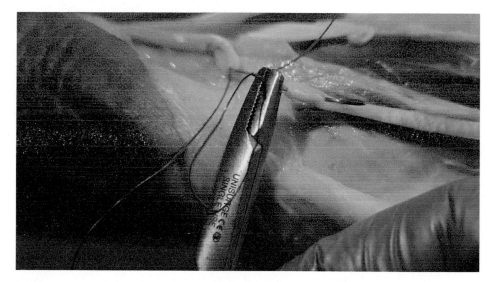

Figure 7.60 Pass the needle down the other cut end.

Much the same as before, take a small perpendicular bite of the tendon, passing the needle towards you.

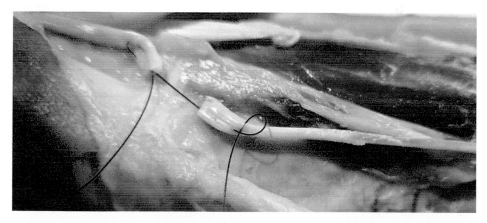

Figure 7.61 Your second anchoring bite complete.

Pass the needle along this half of the tendon, aiming for the middle of the cut end, before passing it along the left half of the tendon, aiming for the side furthest away from you.

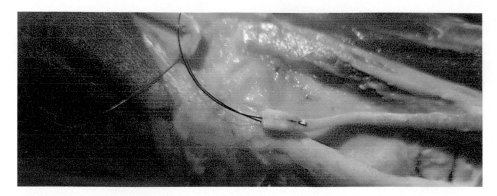

Figure 7.62 Completing the next anchoring bite.

Pass the needle along the left end of the tendon again.

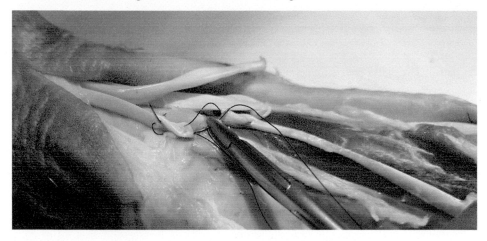

Figure 7.63 Pass the needle along the left end of the tendon again.

Your tendon repair should now be looking like this.

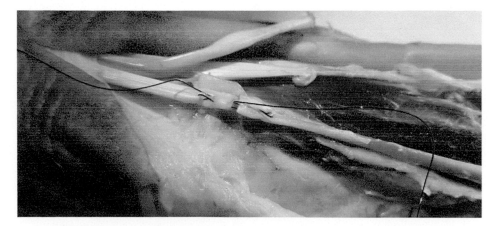

Figure 7.64 Your suture repair at this point.

Much the same as before, take a small perpendicular bite of the tendon, passing the needle away from you.

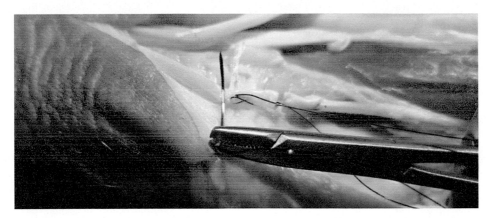

Figure 7.65 The next anchoring bite.

This creates another anchor in the tendon for the repair.

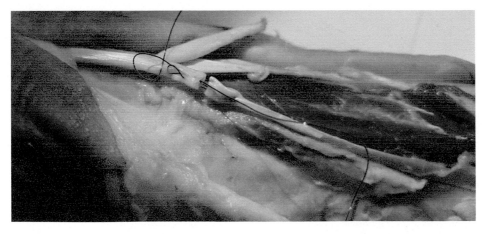

Figure 7.66 The next anchoring bite.

Now pass the needle down the length of the tendon towards the cut end.

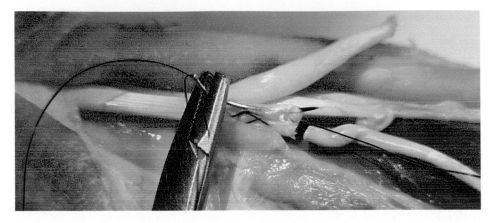

Figure 7.67 Pass the needle down the cut end of the tendon.

Pass the needle down the length of the right-hand side of the cut tendon end.

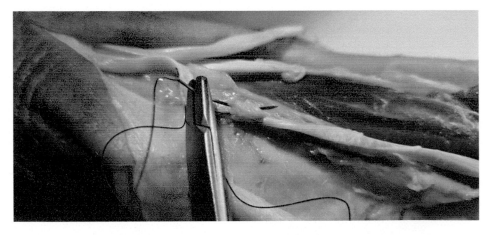

Figure 7.68 Pass the needle down the other cut end of the tendon.

Take a perpendicular bite towards you.

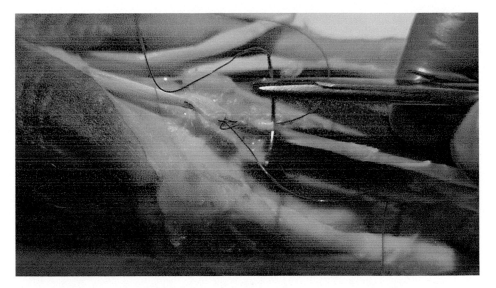

Figure 7.69 Take a perpendicular bite towards you.

Pass the needle back along the cut tendon, aiming for the centre of the cut end. Pull the two suture ends to line up your repair.

Tie this and ensure the knot is buried within the repair.

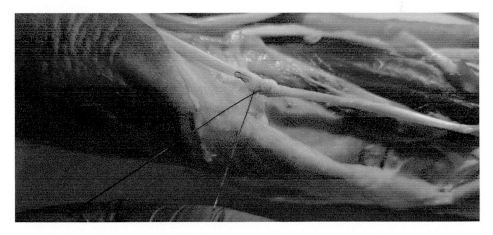

Figure 7.70 Bring the ends together and tie them.

The epitendonous repair

After carrying out your core repair, the next stage is to carry out an epitendonous repair. We will work through a simple continuous suture repair here, but there are many techniques for this.

Start by taking your first bite, trying to keep these bites within the superficial epitendonous layer.

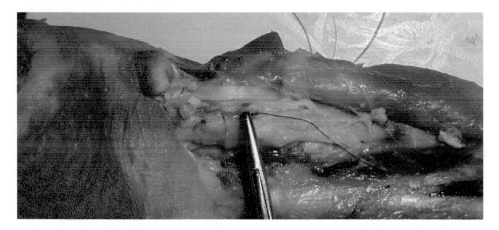

Figure 7.71 Take a superficial bite of the epitendonous layer, crossing the site of the repair.

After pulling through the excess suture, be sure to apply a clip to the free suture end. You will tie onto this at the end.

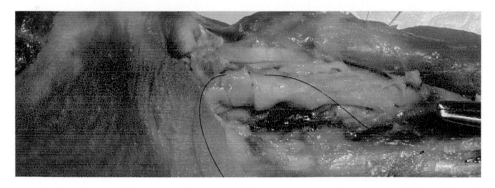

Figure 7.72 Take first bite of the epitendonous layer.

Keep taking epitendonous bites and working around the tendon.

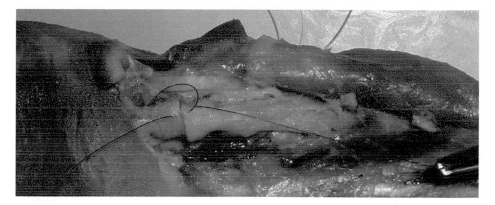

Figure 7.73 Keep taking superficial bites of the epitendonous layer.

Once you have completed the epitendonous repair on the superficial side, you can pass the loose end of the suture under the tendon and use it to partially rotate the tendon.

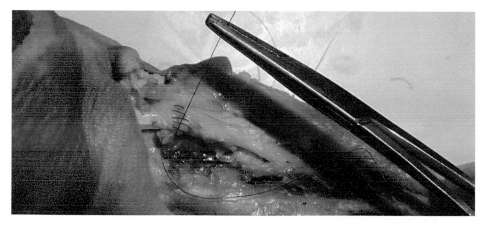

Figure 7.74 Use the ends of the suture to gain access all the way around the tendon.

Once you have carried out the repair all the way around you can now tie onto the loose end to complete the repair. Be sure to bury the knot.

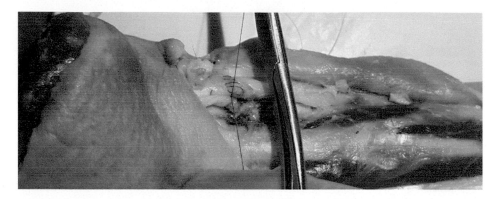

Figure 7.75 Tie your suture ends to complete the epitendonous repair.

This completes a strong and tightly opposed repair.
You should gently test the strength and the glide of the tendon repair.

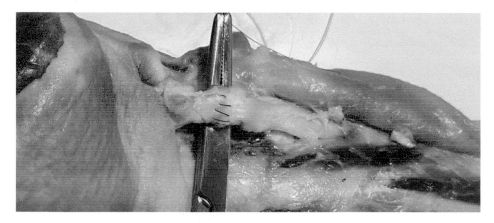

Figure 7.76 Gently test the tensile strength of your repair.

Underrunning a bleeding point (Video 7.7)

Bleeding during surgery can be managed with various techniques, the most basic form of this being the application of pressure and allowing the normal clotting processes to work.

In the next chapter we will discuss diathermy as a haemostasis technique, but sometimes it is necessary to control bleeding by performing a haemostatic suture. This can be a hand tie around a bleeding vessel, or if it is not possible to gain proximal control of the vessel, then the point of bleeding can be compressed with a suture.

The bleeding point is identified and a deep suture passed alongside it.

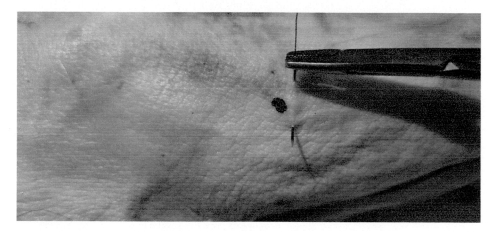

Figure 7.77 Pass your needle alongside the bleeding point.

Then take a second deep pass on the other side of the bleeding point, moving in the same direction as the first bite.

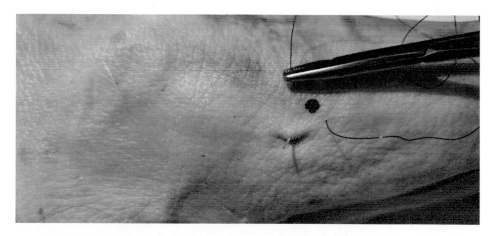

Figure 7.78 Pass your needle alongside the other side of the bleeding point.

This results in a suture that passes over the bleeding point.

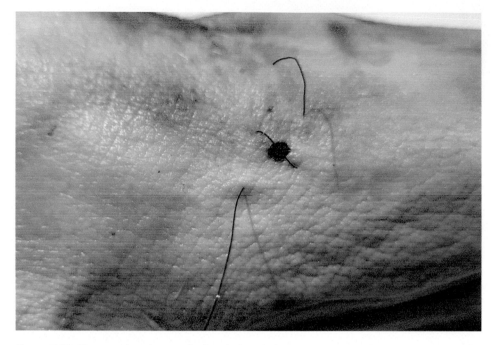

Figure 7.79 The completed suture before being tied.

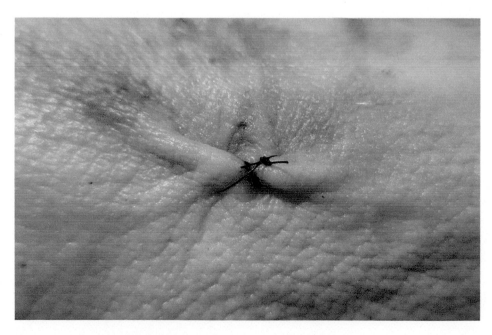

Figure 7.80 The completed suture compressing the bleeding point.

Tying this off then compresses the bleeding point, hopefully with the desired haemostatic effect.

Note

1   Janis, J., 2007. *Essentials of Plastic Surgery*. St. Louis, MO: Quality Medical Pub.

8 Electrosurgery

Graeme M Downes

Principles of electrosurgery

Electrosurgery refers to a group of techniques that utilise an electrical current for the purposes of stopping bleeding or to cut tissues.

In a surgical context this electrical current must operate at high frequency, typically greater than 200 kHz, which avoids neuromuscular stimulation that occurs at lower frequencies such as those found in household circuits.

The waveform of the current will determine what tissue effect occurs. In the simplest form a constant, high-frequency waveform will generate a great deal of heat in the targeted tissue. This results in vaporisation of the tissue, leading to a 'cutting' effect. If the waveform is more intermittent, with infrequent active phases utilising a higher

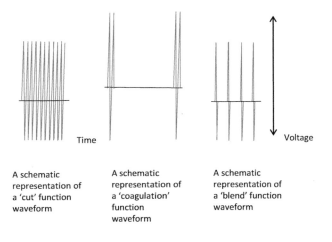

Time

Voltage

A schematic representation of a 'cut' function waveform

A schematic representation of a 'coagulation' function waveform

A schematic representation of a 'blend' function waveform

DOI: 10.1201/b23298-8

voltage, then there will be less heat generated and this results in a 'coagulation' effect. If the cutting effect is comprised of a 100% active phase, then by reducing the active phase there can be a 'blend' function that cuts and coagulates together.

Monopolar and bipolar systems

There are two forms of diathermy in use. The monopolar diathermy system utilises an electrode placed on the patient and the other electrode is the surgical instrument. The other form is bipolar, which utilises a forceps-like instrument that is both electrodes. Functionally this means that the bipolar system only passes current through the tissue being operated on, as opposed to the monopolar system that passes current across the patient.

The advantage of the monopolar system is that the single surgical electrode means that it is possible to use the cut function to dissect tissues, a use that is impractical with a forceps-type instrument.

Principles of patient electrode placement with monopolar diathermy

The site for the patient electrode placement should be unbroken skin, free of hair (shaving is often necessary), with no metallic objects such as joint replacements or old or amateur tattoos. Choose a well-muscled and vascular area, avoiding areas of bony prominence. These measures are intended to maximise the conductive area, dispersing the electrical energy over the whole electrode. Commonly the site chosen will be a lateral thigh or above the hip.

Because the current at the patient electrode is spread over a large plate, there is no heating of the tissues here. Conversely, the current is concentrated at a pointed instrument at the other electrode resulting in a concentration of current and heating.

You should be mindful of other potential risks at the patient electrode, such as the risk of the current diverting along other routes that offer a low resistance path to a grounded connection. This can occur in ECG dots or if the surgical table was damaged and improperly insulated.

Another risk to consider is the use of alcohol-based skin preparations: if these were to pool in between skin creases or the umbilicus then that would represent a fire risk.

The use of monopolar is also contraindicated at distal sites, such as digits, where the current becomes concentrated, potentially resulting in heating of the whole site.

The final and most common consideration with monopolar diathermy is that the current passing through the body is a risk to implanted cardiac or other medical devices. Monopolar should not be used in these cases and bipolar should be used as judiciously as possible.

Risks of surgical smoke

The use of surgical techniques such as diathermy produces smoke which is potentially harmful to the surgical staff. Research has found[1] that surgical smoke contains 95% water vapour and 5% bacterial, viral and cellular debris. In animal models this has been shown to cause inflammatory lung pathology. There have also been multiple carcinogenic compounds identified in surgical smoke.

To ensure risks from surgical smoke are kept as low as possible there should be suction or a bespoke smoke extraction device used alongside diathermy.

Table 8.1 Monopolar summary

Advantages	Disadvantages	Contraindications
Extremely precise, enabling precision dissection	Needs careful placement of patient electrode	Pacemakers, defibrillators (these must be checked before surgery by the cardiac team)
Precise coagulation	Risk of burns if there is an alternative conductive route	Implanted nerve stimulators or drug pumps (such as baclofen)
'Spray' mode enables broad haemostasis	Excessive use can cause skin damage at patient electrode site	

Table 8.2 Bipolar summary

Advantages	Disadvantages	Contraindications
Directs the electrical energy to a specific area	Not able to perform linear cutting actions	Must still be used cautiously when there are implanted medical devices
Lower risk to the patient	Limited special functions	Use of any diathermy directly around a medical device is contraindicated
The prongs of the instrument enable coagulation across small vessels, providing effective ligation		

Note

1 Liu, Y., Song, Y., Hu, X., Yan, L., and Zhu, X. (2019). Awareness of surgical smoke hazards and enhancement of surgical smoke prevention among the gynecologists. *Journal of Cancer*, 10(12), 2788–2799. https://doi.org/10.7150/jca.31464

9 Wound debridement

Graeme M Downes and Rituja Kamble

A dirty, contaminated wound is considered a major reservoir for gross infection and prevents the development of an environment for optimal wound healing. Its primary management is thus a crucial deciding factor in subsequent wound healing. When performed inadequately, the risk of chronic disability secondary to scarring should be remembered.

The videos cited throughout this chapter can be viewed by scanning this QR code.

In this chapter you will learn about:

- The historical context of debridement
- Key considerations of the procedure
- How to perform wound debridement
- Key considerations following the procedure
- Advice from the clinical setting

DOI: 10.1201/b23298-9

One of the first proponents of early and through debridement of traumatic wounds was the French surgeon Dominique Jean Larrey (1766–1842). Working as a surgeon in Napoleon's army, Larrey advocated the surgical 'unbridling' of wounds – the French term being *'débrider'*, from which we get the word debridement. This focus on surgical decontamination of wounds was carried forward by Karl Von Reyher (1786–1857), a Prussian military surgeon[1]. This prompt removal of dead and non-viable tissue cleans wounds and removes material that will become nothing more than a bacterial growth medium.

In a time before antibiotics, this aggressive management of wounds was the most effective method at reducing the rates of devastating wound infections, and in the modern era the use of debridement remains a crucial component of managing traumatic and infected wounds.

Wound debridement (Video 9.1)

Debriding a wound

The key considerations with wound debridement are as follows:

- Removal of any debris or foreign material. This is crucial to enable proper healing and remove contamination. Where the foreign material is radio opaque, X-ray can be utilised to identify the extent of contamination.

- Dead tissue can then be identified; non-viable skin will lack a capillary refill and will not bleed when cut. Non-viable skin should be cut away until viable tissue is reached. Any attempt to close dead skin is likely to lead to difficult wound healing and dehiscence. Non-viable fat will be loose and can be wiped away. Non-viable muscle will be grey and will not fasciculate when stimulated, nor will it bleed when cut.

- Any potentially non-viable bone, nerve or vasculature should only be debrided with specialist advice.

- After completing all debridement, the wound should be heavily irrigated with warmed saline. Depending on the size of the wound this may require large volumes of fluid (1–3 litres is usually sensible).

- The wound should be dressed with consideration for adequate coverage and to allowing further inspection to occur.

Here we have a heavily contaminated wound, with non-viable tissue indicated by the black colouration.

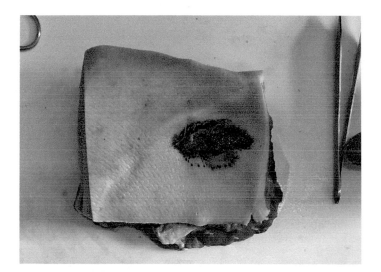

Figure 9.1 A contaminated wound.

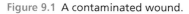

The first step is to explore the wound with your instruments, ensuring that you do not probe with your fingers if there is any risk of sharp foreign material. Avoid using your blade to cut through structures at this stage and try to use dissecting scissors and forceps to probe and manipulate the tissue. Any contaminants should be removed.

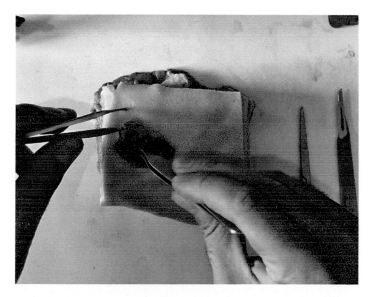

Figure 9.2 Removing foreign material contamination.

The skin edges should be investigated and assessed for viability; any non-viable tissue should be excised with a scalpel. It is important to do this conservatively to avoid over-excision of viable tissue.

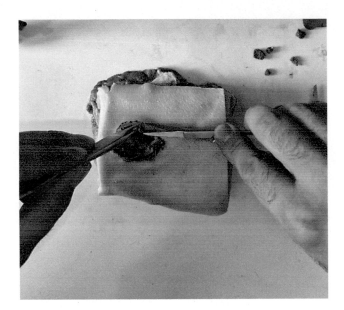

Figure 9.3 Skin edges being debrided.

After removing any dead skin, the deeper layers should be investigated, and minimal muscle debridement carried out if indicated.

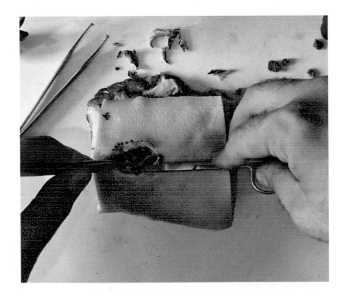

Figure 9.4 Non-viable muscle being debrided.

Once all the non-viable tissue is removed, the wound can be explored again to look for any key structures that may have been damaged.

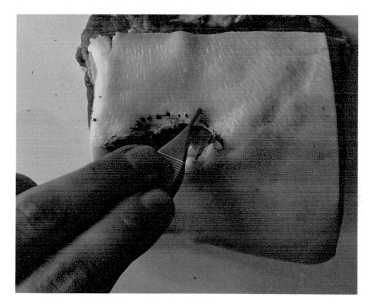

Figure 9.5 Exploring the wound.

Finally, the wound can be thoroughly irrigated and dressed appropriately.

After debridement

After debriding a wound, a decision should be made about the approach to closure. For a contaminated or infected wound, primary closure is unlikely to be advisable as this will risk creating an abscess. Instead, these soiled wounds are likely to benefit from a delayed primary closure, often utilising a negative pressure dressing, or healing by secondary intention with dressing care.

Such dressing care for wounds that are healing by secondary intention will focus on preventing premature epidermal closure. This will use packing dressings to allow wounds to granulate from the base upwards.

For contaminated wounds, antibiotic therapy is usually indicated, based on local guidelines.

Negative pressure wound therapy

There are various commercial devices that can be used to create a sub-atmospheric wound environment, and this is widely regarded as beneficial for wound healing.

It is postulated[2] that this environment has four beneficial effects on wound healing:

1. Wound contraction due to the physical action of the vacuum reduces the size of the defect and the dead space.

2. On a microscopic level, the vacuum forces are believed to promote cell differentiation and inflammatory modulation. The interface between the porous sponge dressing of typical systems further contributes to mechanical strain on tissues that is expected to promote healing through a proliferation response to growth factors. This microstrain promotes angiogenesis and tissue growth.[3]

3. Fluid removal by the vacuum reduces shearing forces on the newly forming tissue and reduces the bacterial load within the wound.

4. The vacuum has the additional benefit of optimising the wound environment, ensuring a suitable level of moisture and thermoregulation. It also allows for the removal of extracellular fluid that could hamper healing.

Advice from the clinical setting

The context of a dirty, contaminated wound is important when considering the steps and timing of its management. In particular, it is important to ascertain key factors from the history, examination and investigations:

● Is the wound contaminated with marine, sewage or agricultural waste?

● Is the wound eroding into a joint?

● Is the wound secondary to an animal or human bite?

● Is there a concurrent underlying fracture?

The presence of any of these should prompt urgent senior escalation and timely action to debride, irrigate and prevent the spread of potential infection. Where possible, local and national guidelines should be consulted and adhered to.

Notes

1 Le Vay, D., 1974. Larrey and debridement. *BMJ*, 4(5943), pp. 531–531.
2 Huang, C., Leavitt, T., Bayer, L., and Orgill, D., 2014. Effect of negative pressure wound therapy on wound healing. *Current Problems in Surgery*, 51(7), pp. 301–331.
3 Janis, J., 2007. *Essentials of Plastic Surgery*. St. Louis, MO: Quality Medical Pub. pp. 121–125.

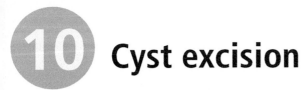

10 Cyst excision

Graeme M Downes and Rituja Kamble

Overview of common cysts

The videos cited throughout this chapter can be viewed by scanning this QR code.

Derived from the Greek term *'kustis'*, meaning 'bladder', a cyst is defined as an abnormal membranous sac containing gas, liquid or semi-solid material. True cysts have a wall comprised of epithelium[1]. They can occur in any tissue type and are of varying aetiology. The first types of cyst requiring excision that you will encounter in your surgical career are likely to be those arising from the skin, so we will focus on these.

In this chapter you will learn about:

● Commonly encountered types of cysts

● How to assess a cyst

● How to excise a cyst

● Common pitfalls

Epidermoid cysts

These are extremely common and generally considered to be benign, but recent evidence suggests that they can undergo malignant transformation[2]. They can occur on any skin,

DOI: 10.1201/b23298-10

but most commonly on the face, neck and trunk, and are often referred to as sebaceous cysts although they do not have an association with sebaceous glands.

They are lined with stratified squamous epithelium which leads to the accumulation of keratin within the dermis or subepidermal layer, and usually present with a punctum communicating to the skin surface.

Epidermal cysts present as mobile nodules with a central punctum.

They usually occur spontaneously but can also follow trauma. This occurs when a traumatic injury results in the inoculation of epidermis into the dermis, where the epidermis continues to produce keratin forming a cyst, often referred to as an epidermal inclusion cyst. This can also occur from an iatrogenic cause where epidermis is buried under dermis during wound closure, and should be judiciously avoided.

Pilar cysts

These are a rarer type of skin cyst arising from the root sheath of a hair follicle that occurs when there is an accumulation of keratin in the follicle[3]. They are, therefore, intradermal cysts and are lined with stratified squamous epithelium. They are also referred to as trichilemmal cysts and are most commonly found on the scalp. Rarely, they can undergo malignant transformation and are then referred to as proliferating trichilemmal cysts.

Pilar cysts commonly present as well-circumscribed, smooth, firm and mobile nodules. Note that they have no central punctum.

Abscess

Following trauma, such as a penetrating injury, infection can occur within the deeper structures of the skin. If this fails to resolve, then a collection of cellular debris, fluid and pus can form within the skin leading to an abscess. These will be differentiated from cysts by the history, where there will be a short history of rapid growth, pain, erythema and possible systemic symptoms.

Other cysts

There are a wide variety of other true cysts and pseudocysts, some of which are best managed with surgical excision. However, the wide variety of management options and specialist nature of these cysts make them less suitable for discussing in this book.

Assessment of a cyst

After taking a history and gaining consent, you should wash your hands and systematically examine the lump. A suggested format is as follows:

Site – location of the lump in relation to anatomical landmarks. Then further examination in order to ascertain the lump's relation to the surrounding structures. You may be able to identify what plane the lump exists in, and if it is adherent to nerve, tendon or bone.

Size – measured accurately in two or three dimensions.

Shape – is it a regular shape, such as a sphere or ovoid, or something irregular?

Surface – are there skin changes, such as erythema, warmth, any skin damage, punctum? Any colour changes?

Consistency – generally described as hard, firm or soft. These can be equated to hard being like the bridge of your nose, firm like the tip of your nose or soft like your cheek.

Pulsatile – is there a vascular thrill to the lump, strongly suggestive of an aneurysm or vascular malformation?

Reducible – can the lump be reduced or compressed? Suggestive of a vascular malformation or a hernia, respectively.

Fluctuation – does percussion or balloting of the lump transmit through the lump? This suggests a fluid or semi-fluid consistency.

Mobility – is the lump mobile in the tissue? Does it move with muscular contraction? Does it move with the dragging of overlying skin? This all gives valuable information on the likely origin of the lump.

Transillumination – shining a pen torch into the lump may light it up brilliantly, which would suggest that it is fluid filled.

Blood tests and imaging, such as ultrasound, may be useful adjuncts to complete your examination and aid diagnosis.

Excision of a cyst (Video 10.1)

Once the diagnosis has been made and a decision taken to proceed to surgery, then the lump should be excised.

What follows is a stepwise example of the excision of a simulated cyst.

It is important that the skin lesion should be marked with a surgical marker pen before any infiltration of local anaesthesia. This is crucial as the volume of the local anaesthetic will make palpation of the cyst very difficult and the restoration of the skin anatomy more difficult.

Below is the tissue containing a cyst that has been marked with the outline of the palpable lump, the punctum and a planned excision of an ellipse of skin to remove the punctum and allow access to dissect out the cyst. By excising an ellipse of skin this will reduce the anatomical dead space once the cyst is removed and reduce the risk of seroma, abscess or recurrence.

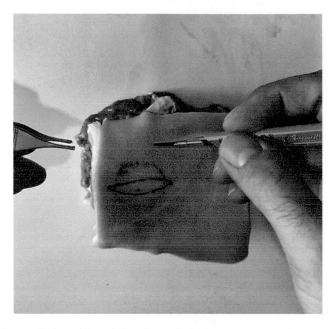

Figure 10.1 The surgical marking of the planned excision.

Start by cutting along your marked incision down to the dermis. When excising an epidermoid cyst by incorporating the punctum in your skin ellipse, you will often find that the cyst is tethered to this piece of skin. This will enable you to manipulate this skin piece to gain better access to the cyst for dissection.

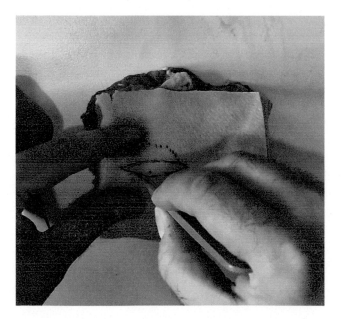

Figure 10.2 Incision of the skin ellipse.

Once you have completed your skin incision, you should proceed with completing the incision at one corner. This will enable you to lift the skin ellipse to begin getting around the cyst below.

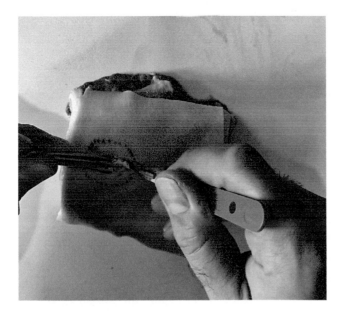

Figure 10.3 Lifting the excised skin ellipse.

In this example the cyst is not adherent to the skin so the next step is to completely remove the skin ellipse to gain adequate exposure to the underlying cyst. Note: this can often be a difficult step, as removing the ellipse in too deep a layer may risk puncturing the cyst.

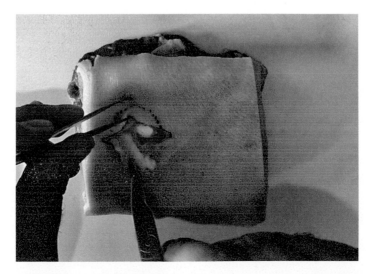

Figure 10.4 Completing the skin excision.

Now that there is good exposure of the cyst it can be manipulated and freed from any adhesions. At this point a small self-retractor, such as an Alms, would be useful. It is preferable to use curved dissecting scissors for this step. This is to spread apart the tissues and further prevent puncturing the cyst.

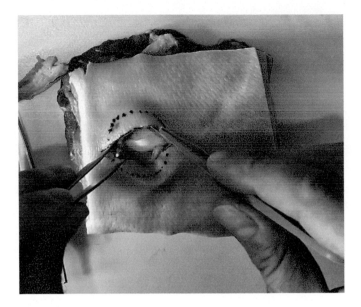

Figure 10.5 Exposing and dissecting out the cyst.

Once free the cyst can be removed, and the defect thoroughly washed with normal saline. It is preferable if the cyst can be removed with the sac intact as this will minimize contamination and leaving behind any sac will significantly increase the chance of recurrence.

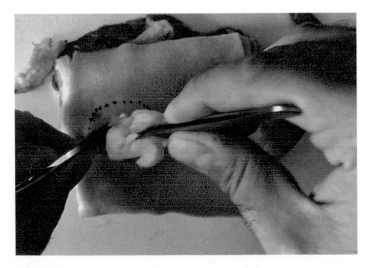

Figure 10.6 Removing the cyst and the sac.

After the removal of the cyst and the washing of the cavity the wound can now be closed. The elliptical excision should enable the skin to be closed with a neat linear scar. Deep dermal followed by epidermal closure is preferable.

The cyst should be sent for histology to confirm the diagnosis and ensure this is not a malignant or concerning diagnosis.

Common pitfalls

The most common pitfall is puncturing the cyst and causing it to rupture intra-operatively. In some cases, this might be unavoidable, but for the most part this can be prevented by:

● Avoiding deep structures when removing the overlying ellipse of skin.

● Using dissecting scissors to spread apart tissues when removing the cyst and avoiding cutting towards the cyst.

● Not gripping the cyst too forcefully with your forceps. Attempt to grip the overlying lining of the cyst where possible.

The other common pitfall is incomplete removal of the cyst which may occur during difficult dissections when part of the cyst lining is left behind. This results in a very high likelihood that the cyst will recur and could be avoided by careful dissection of the tissue plane inferior to the cyst prior to excising it.

Notes

1 Hoang, V.T., Trinh, C.T., Nguyen, C.H., Chansomphou, V., Chansomphou, V., and Tran, T.T.T., 2019. Overview of epidermoid cyst. *European Journal of Radiology Open*, 5(6), pp. 291–301. doi: 10.1016/j.ejro.2019.08.003. PMID: 31516916; PMCID: PMC6732711.

2 Zito, P.M. and Scharf, R., *Epidermoid Cyst*. [Updated 2022 Jul 10]. In: StatPearls [Internet]. Treasure Island (FL): StatPearls Publishing; 2022 Jan. Available from: https://www.ncbi. nlm.nih.gov/books/NBK499974

3 Varghese, R., Yabit, F., Alrifai, A., et al., April 07, 2022. Pilar cysts of the head and neck: A case report. *Cureus*, 14(4), e23932. doi:10.7759/cureus.23932

11 Making the most of your surgical placement

Howard Chu

Introduction

Pursuing a career in surgery requires you to be committed, enthusiastic and dedicated. The training pathway is long and there is strong competition to progress. It is important to be well motivated to approach these challenges and to keep pursuing your goal to become a surgeon.

There are specific challenges to progressing through the different stages of surgical training and it is advisable to be aware of what is required at each stage so that you can plan when to undertake the various courses, projects and exams, rather than trying to accomplish these in a time-pressured way. In this chapter we will cover the different considerations at medical school, in the foundation years, during Core Surgical Training and looking to be successful in securing a place on Higher Surgical Training.

Broadly speaking, undertakings such as higher degrees, membership exams, teaching experience and research will take the longest time to achieve. It is certainly sensible to start thinking about these aspects of your portfolio and to plan when will be a good time for you to focus on these aspects.

Medical school

Making a career choice in surgery can be daunting, so early planning and strategizing will allow you to maximise every opportunity and tailor your curriculum vitae towards this goal.

During your surgery placements at medical school, embed yourself within the unit and get involved with projects. It would be ideal to choose projects that you can

DOI: 10.1201/b23298-11

contribute to comfortably and take the chance to present these at a national or international level. Many institutions, such as the Royal Society of Medicine (RSM) and the Association of Surgeons In Training (ASIT), offer the opportunity to submit work by students for national presentations and potential prizes. By maximising attendance in theatre and clinics you will gain a basic understanding of what the speciality involves.

If there is a university surgical society that offers basic surgical skills training, then use this to gain experience and build your leadership skills through a committee role.

There are numerous conferences that are aimed towards undergraduates, for example those run by specialist organisations such as BAPRAS, BOA, ASIT and RSM. This is a great place to network with other students, present your work and talk to consultants within this field. These opportunities for networking can open up potential avenues for becoming involved in projects or undertaking student selected modules or taster weeks.

Foundation years

During this time, it is recommended you focus upon gaining the skills required as a foundation doctor. It can be a tough time acclimatising to the peaks and troughs of doctor life. By attending theatre lists you can gain basic surgical skills, like knot tying and suturing, whilst also understanding the patient's journey. Towards the end of Year 1 you should start thinking about applying for core training and consider a themed job in your preferred speciality (if you have decided) to best maximise training.

Make sure you use your full study budget – attendance on courses such as Basic Surgical Skills, Advance Trauma Life Support, and Care of the Critically Ill Surgical Patient are all very beneficial. Note that being in date for a trauma course is a requirement to complete Core Surgical Training and currently places on these courses are difficult to find, so if you have a chance to attend a trauma course it should certainly be considered.

Foundation years are also a good time to find opportunities to expand your leadership experience. You will gain valuable experience and confidence as well as much needed points for applications by taking on such local roles, such as doctors' mess representatives; regional roles, such as being a foundation doctor representative; or national roles, if you can find the opportunities.

Core Surgical Training

Core Surgical Training (CST) can be a hectic two years whilst trying to gain the MRCS, starting to perform basic procedures and think about applying for national training. If you have the capacity to do so – or if you take time out after foundation – then consider undertaking your MRCS before CST. This will free up some of your focus during CST to prioritise the practical training.

If you have a definite idea of what speciality you wish to pursue, try to maximise as much time as you can in that speciality. Often other colleagues would be happy to switch placements, though this will be at the discretion of your training programme director (TPD). But if you only have a short stint within your chosen speciality, then maximise your opportunities during other placements – for example, there is overlap between hand surgery performed in Orthopaedic and Plastic Surgery units.

Even if you are not able to change placements you can always work with your colleagues to gain the best exposure. It may be that there is a particular case that you would benefit from being involved in and there may be the possibility to come to an agreement with a colleague. It may be that, for example, they could cover your ward commitment and you can do the same for them in return.

Do not forget that you can always continue projects with your chosen team and ask to attend lists or clinics within your free study periods.

To ensure that you maximise your training on theatre lists, always see what is on the list beforehand and – if you have the opportunity – go through the case with the registrar or consultant allocated to the list. If you are able to find out what cases are on the list early enough, then you can look through the stages of the operation and the relevant anatomy in advance. You can always ask whether there are parts of the operation that you could perform whilst supervised.

Arriving early before the team does always sets a good example. It is also nice to speak to the patient beforehand so you can understand first-hand the journey they have taken up to this point. Read through their notes and look up any relevant histology or blood results.

When you start in your surgical placement, look to gain enough experience and knowledge to take part in the consenting process. Initially you can complete the consent form to the best of your ability and then have this reviewed by someone more senior. As you gain more experience, you will be able to fully complete and take valid consent for the more common procedures.

During the operation engage with the team and ask questions. Offer to close the wound as this will be your chance to refine this skill. Closing the wound is often the first part of the operation that you will be able to perform under supervision – utilising resources such as this book and attending courses will help you to be as well prepared for this as possible.

If you come across any interesting cases or projects, take the opportunity to approach the team to see if you can lead on writing this up or act as the principal investigator. Case studies are some of the most straightforward projects to write up, but the number of journals that will publish these without payment is limited. Letters and abstracts are another option for more straightforward publications.

Conclusion

Be aware of the scoring criteria for CST and Higher Surgical Training applications and have a plan for what you are going to aim to achieve and when you will do this. Experience of teaching, leadership, research and audit, as well as gaining higher qualifications are usually scoring areas. Alongside this, take every chance to maximise your exposure to surgical specialties and improve your knowledge and surgical skills.

With good preparation and planning you can make yourself a strong candidate for competitive surgical training positions and progress towards your goals.

Appendix 1
Suturing checklist

Rituja Kamble and Graeme M Downes

To aid you during on-call shifts we have prepared a checklist of all the equipment you will need to suture a wound, so you can refer to this when needed.

Before suturing a wound, you should consider the steps involved in the procedure and which of these steps will be performed in a sterile field:

1. Preparing and cleaning the wound (Non-sterile)
2. Wound closure (Sterile)
3. Dressing the wound (Sterile)

You can then consider what equipment is needed in each field.

1. Preparing and cleaning the wound (Non-sterile)
   - Inco pad
   - Light source
   - Apron/gown
   - Non-sterile gloves
   - Local anaesthetic preparation
   - Syringe
   - Drawing-up needle – ensure it is filtered if using glass vials
   - Injecting needle – a 23 g (blue) or 25 g (orange) needle is usually appropriate
   - Gauze
   - Sharps bin
   - Sterile bowl
   - Skin/wound cleaning – povodene-iodine, saline or similar. Avoid chlorhexidine on open wounds
2. Wound closure (Sterile)
   - A minor ops pack including:
     - Needle holders
     - Forceps (toothed and non-toothed as needed)
     - Scissors
     - Sterile gauze – at least 10 pieces
     - A sterile drape
     - Container, such as a kidney dish, for scrub solution

- An appropriate suture
- Sterile gloves

3. Dressing the wound (Sterile)
    - Dressing – semi occlusive dressing or non-adherent dressing and bandage depending on the size and contour of the wound

Appendix 2
Advice after sutures

Graeme M Downes

After having stitches, also known as sutures, you will need to ensure that they are kept clean and dry.

You should also look out for any signs of infection and seek advice straightaway if you are worried.

Protecting your stitches

- Do not get them wet

- Avoid picking or scratching at the stitches

- Avoid strenuous activity that might break the stitches

- Avoid getting them dirty – activities such as gardening and DIY should be avoided while your wound is healing

Signs of infection

- Increasing pain

- Increasing swelling

- Redness

- Heat

- Bleeding

- Pus coming from the wound

- Any smell

- Any fever

- Swollen glands in your armpit, neck or groin

When to remove your stitches

Your surgeon should have told you if you have absorbable or non-absorbable stitches. The absorbable kind will not need any removal.

If you have non-absorbable stitches, then these should be removed at the following times.

- On the face or head: 5–7 days

- Areas of high stress: 14 days

- Other areas: 10–14 days

If you have any immediate concerns then contact 111, your GP or the accident and emergency department. Advice can also be sought from the team that carried out your procedure.

Index